Health Effects of Ingested Fluoride

Subcommittee on Health Effects of Ingested Fluoride

Committee on Toxicology
Board on Environmental Studies and Toxicology
Commission on Life Sciences
National Research Council

NATIONAL ACADEMY PRESS
Washington, D.C.   1993

NATIONAL ACADEMY PRESS 2101 Constitution Ave., N.W., Washington, D.C. 20418

NOTICE: The project that is the subject of this report was approved by the Governing Board of the National Research Council, whose members are drawn from the councils of the National Academy of Sciences, the National Academy of Engineering, and the Institute of Medicine. The members of the committee responsible for the report were chosen for their special competencies and with regard for appropriate balance.

This report has been reviewed by a group other than the authors according to procedures approved by a Report Review Committee consisting of members of the National Academy of Sciences, the National Academy of Engineering, and the Institute of Medicine.

The National Academy of Sciences is a private, non-profit, self-perpetuating society of distinguished scholars engaged in scientific and engineering research, dedicated to the furtherance of science and technology and to their use for the general welfare. Upon the authority of the charter granted to it by the Congress in 1863, the Academy has a mandate that requires it to advise the federal government on scientific and technical matters. Dr. Frank Press is president of the National Academy of Sciences.

The National Academy of Engineering was established in 1964, under the charter of the National Academy of Sciences, as a parallel organization of outstanding engineers. It is autonomous in its administration and in the selection of its members, sharing with the National Academy of Sciences the responsibility for advising the federal government. The National Academy of Engineering also sponsors engineering programs aimed at meeting national needs, encourages education and research, and recognizes the superior achievements of engineers. Dr. Robert M. White is president of the National Academy of Engineering.

The Institute of Medicine was established in 1970 by the National Academy of Sciences to secure the services of eminent members of appropriate professions in the examination of policy matters pertaining to the health of the public. The Institute acts under the responsibility given to the National Academy of Sciences by its congressional charter to be an adviser to the federal government and, upon its own initiative, to identify issues of medical care, research, and education. Dr. Kenneth I. Shine is president of the Institute of Medicine.

The National Research Council was organized by the National Academy of Sciences in 1916 to associate the broad community of science and technology with the Academy's purposes of furthering knowledge and advising the federal government. Functioning in accordance with general policies determined by the Academy, the Council has become the principal operating agency of both the National Academy of Sciences and the National Academy of Engineering in providing services to the government, the public, and the scientific and engineering communities. The Council is administered jointly by both Academies and the Institute of Medicine. Dr. Frank Press and Dr. Robert M. White are chairman and vice chairman, respectively, of the National Research Council.

The project was supported by U.S. Environmental Protection Agency Contract CR-819504-01-0.

Library of Congress Catalog Card No. 93-85306
International Standard Book No. 0-309-04975-X

Additional copies of this report are available from: National Academy Press, 2101 Constitution Avenue, NW, Box 285, Washington, DC 20055.

B-186

Printed in the United States of America

First Printing, August 1993
Second Printing, March 1995

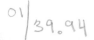

SUBCOMMITTEE ON HEALTH EFFECTS OF INGESTED FLUORIDE

BERNARD M. WAGNER *(Chair)*, Wagner Associates, Inc., Millburn, N.J.
BRIAN A. BURT, University of Michigan, Ann Arbor, Mich.
KENNETH P. CANTOR, National Cancer Institute, Rockville, Md.
DANIEL KREWSKI, Health & Welfare Canada, Ottawa, Ontario
STEVEN M. LEVY, University of Iowa, Iowa City, Iowa
ERNEST EUGENE McCONNELL, Raleigh, N.C.
GARY M. WHITFORD, Medical College of Georgia, Augusta, Ga.

Staff

RICHARD D. THOMAS, Program Director
KULBIR S. BAKSHI, Project Director
RUTH E. CROSSGROVE, Editor
CATHERINE M. KUBIK, Senior Program Assistant
RUTH P. DANOFF, Project Assistant

COMMITTEE ON TOXICOLOGY

Board on Environmental Studies and Toxicology

COMMISSION ON LIFE SCIENCES

Other Recent Reports of The Board on Environmental Studies and Toxicology

Pesticides in the Diets of Infants and Children (1993)
Issues in Risk Assessment (1993)
Setting Priorities for Land Conservation (1993)
Protecting Visibility in National Parks and Wilderness Areas (1993)
Biologic Markers in Immunotoxicology (1992)
Dolphins and the Tuna Industry (1992)
Environmental Neurotoxicology (1992)
Hazardous Materials on the Public Lands (1992)
Science and the National Parks (1992)
Animals as Sentinels of Environmental Health Hazards (1991)
Assessment of the U.S. Outer Continental Shelf Environmental Studies
    Program, Volumes I-IV (1991-1993)
Human Exposure Assessment for Airborne Pollutants (1991)
Monitoring Human Tissues for Toxic Substances (1991)
Rethinking the Ozone Problem in Urban and Regional Air Pollution
    (1991)
Decline of the Sea Turtles (1990)
Tracking Toxic Substances at Industrial Facilities (1990)
Biologic Markers in Pulmonary Toxicology (1989)
Biologic Markers in Reproductive Toxicology (1989)

Copies of these reports may be ordered from
the National Academy Press
(800) 624-6242
(202) 334-3313

PREFACE

Fluoridation of public water supplies has aroused considerable discussion among scientists and the general public since it began in 1945. Although the majority of scientists support the measure, some take the view that fluoridation can produce not only adverse cosmetic effects from severe dental fluorosis, but also adverse health effects.

Scientists have become increasingly aware of the potential for exposure to toxic concentrations of fluoride from water and other sources (e.g., foods, processed beverages, dental products, and fluoride supplements). Thus, accurate information on the potential health effects of fluoride is needed. To address that need, the U.S. Environmental Protection Agency (EPA) requested that the Committee on Toxicology (COT) review the health effects of ingested fluoride and determine whether EPA's maximum contaminant level of 4 milligrams (mg) of fluoride per liter (L) of drinking water is appropriate. In response, COT organized the Subcommittee on Health Effects of Ingested Fluoride, which included scientists with expertise in toxicology, pathology, medicine, dentistry, epidemiology, biostatistics, and risk assessment. The subcommittee reviewed various kinds of toxicity that have been attributed to ingestion of fluoride (dental fluorosis; bone fracture; reproductive, renal, gastrointestinal, and immunological toxicities; genotoxicity; and carcinogenicity) and assessed the current EPA drinking-water standard for fluoride to determine if it is protective of public health. The report of the subcommittee is intended for use by EPA in deciding whether to maintain or revise its current drinking-water standard for fluoride.

xiii

The subcommittee gratefully acknowledges the interest and support of Edward Ohanian and Kenneth Bailey of EPA. We also thank other persons who provided information or prepared presentations for the subcommittee, including Steven Gordon, National Institutes of Health; Daniel Hoffman, George Washington University; Lent Johnson, John Pletcher, and Michael Slayter, Armed Forces Institute of Pathology; and Frank Young, U.S. Department of Health and Human Services. We are grateful to the anonymous reviewers for their many helpful comments and suggestions that have resulted in improvements in the presentation of the subcommittee's findings.

This report could not have been produced without the untiring efforts of the National Research Council staff: Richard D. Thomas, program director; Ruth E. Crossgrove, editor; Ruth Danoff, project assistant; and Catherine Kubik, senior program assistant.

Finally, the subcommittee gratefully acknowledges the persistence, patience, and expertise of Kulbir S. Bakshi, project director of the subcommittee, in bringing this report to its final form.

Bernard Wagner, *Chair*
Subcommittee on Health Effects
of Ingested Fluoride

Rogene F. Henderson, *Chair*
Committee on Toxicology

CONTENTS

xv

HEALTH EFFECTS OF INGESTED FLUORIDE

EXECUTIVE SUMMARY

INTRODUCTION

Fluoridation of drinking water has been a subject of controversy for decades. Over the past 50 years, the incidence of dental caries (cavities) has declined considerably in the United States, an important health advance that most scientists attribute principally to increased access to fluoridated water and dental products. According to the U.S. Centers for Disease Control and Prevention, approximately 132 million Americans now receive drinking water that contains fluoride, either naturally occurring or added, at concentrations of 0.7 milligrams per liter (mg/L) or higher. Since the 1960s, the U.S. Public Health Service (PHS) has recommended an "optimal" fluoride concentration of 0.7-1.2 mg/L to prevent dental caries and minimize dental fluorosis. However, there has been an increase in the prevalence of dental fluorosis a mottling of tooth enamel that ranges from barely discernible enamel flecks in its mildest forms to staining and pitting in its severest forms; the severest forms are rare in the United States. EPA considers dental fluorosis to be a cosmetic effect and not an adverse health effect.

Recent findings have renewed longstanding concerns of those who oppose water fluoridation, claiming that ingestion of fluoride can lead to a variety of unwanted effects. One animal study reported an equivocal increase in osteosarcomas (malignant bone tumors) in male rats, but not in female rats, at very high concentrations (100-175 mg/L). However, that result was not substantiated in a subsequent study in rats at even higher doses.

In the United States, a few cases of crippling skeletal fluorosis (an increase in the thickness of bones, which in advanced stages, is associated with decreased mobility of joints and pain) have been reported in humans only when fluoride concentrations in drinking water exceeded 8 mg/L over many years. That concentration is much higher than the PHS recommendation of 0.7-1.2 mg/L. To prevent skeletal fluorosis, the U.S. Environmental Protection Agency (EPA) set the maximum contaminant level (MCL) for fluoride at 4 mg/L of drinking water. In addition to fluoride in drinking water, however, people also can ingest fluoride in toothpaste, mouth rinse, and dietary fluoride supplements or in beverages and foods prepared with fluoridated water. As a result, many Americans might ingest more "incidental" fluoride than was anticipated by PHS and EPA in recommending standards for drinking water.

EPA responded to the concerns by requesting that the National Research Council's Board on Environmental Studies and Toxicology (BEST) review the current toxicological and exposure data on fluoride and determine whether EPA's current MCL of 4 mg/L is acceptable for protecting the public from potential adverse health effects of fluoride. EPA also asked BEST to identify gaps in the fluoride toxicity data and to make recommendations for future research.

In response to EPA's request, BEST's Committee on Toxicology established the Subcommittee on Health Effects of Ingested Fluoride. The subcommittee based its evaluation on a detailed examination of current data in the following areas:

- Intake, metabolism, and disposition of fluoride.
- Dental fluorosis.
- Bone strength and the risk of bone fracture.
- Effects on the renal, gastrointestinal, and immune systems.
- Reproductive effects in animals.
- Genotoxicity.
- Carcinogenicity in animals and humans.

This report deals with the possible toxic effects of ingested fluoride in humans. It does not attempt to weigh fluoride's well-documented health benefits against its possible adverse health effects.

INTAKE, METABOLISM, AND DISPOSITION OF FLUORIDE

The major sources of fluoride intake are water and other beverages, food, and fluoride-containing dental products. Groundwater, a major source of drinking water in many communities, can contain fluoride at concentrations ranging from less than 0.1 mg/L to more than 100 mg/L in some parts of the world (e.g., Africa and China). Coffee, tea, and soft drinks made with that water might have corresponding concentrations of fluoride. Concentrations in food depend on the levels in the soil, but they can increase or decrease depending on the fluoride concentrations in the water used in food preparation. Dental products available in the United States and meant to be used topically (and not ingested) contain fluoride at concentrations ranging from 230 to over 12,000 parts per million (ppm).

The average intake of dietary fluoride by young children whose water supply contains fluoride at 0.7-1.2 mg/L is approximately 0.5 mg per day, although substantial variation occurs. Because it is associated with optimal fluoridation, this level of fluoride intake (0.5 mg per day, or 0.04-0.07 mg per kilogram (kg) of body weight per day) generally has also been accepted as optimal. Nursing infants receive negligible fluoride from breast milk, but intake from formulas can range from less than 0.4 to over 1.0 mg per day when reconstituting powder concentrate with fluoridated water, a range that can exceed the optimal level. Dietary intake by adults in areas with fluoridated water has been estimated at 1.2-2.2 mg per day, although intake by some individuals, such as outdoor laborers in warm climates or those with urinary disorders, can be considerably higher.

Accurate estimates of fluoride exposure cannot be based simply on the concentration of fluoride in drinking water. For example, dental products can be an important source of ingested fluoride, especially for young children who have poor control over the swallowing reflex. Even for older children, intake from toothpaste and mouth rinse can still equal the daily intake from food, water, and other beverages. Soft drinks, which often contain fluoride at 0.3-0.5 mg per 12-ounce serving, are an important additional source of fluoride. Studies of dental fluorosis indicate that children's exposure to fluoride has increased since the 1970s.

Approximately 75-90% of the fluoride ingested each day is absorbed from the alimentary tract. Because of its chemical affinity for calcium compounds, about half of that fluoride becomes associated with teeth and bones within 24 hours of ingestion. In growing children, even more of the ingested fluoride is retained because of the large surface area provided by numerous and loosely organized bone crystallites. The remaining fluoride is eliminated almost exclusively by the kidneys, and the rate of renal clearance is directly related to urinary pH. As a result, diet, drugs, metabolism, and other factors can affect the extent to which fluoride is retained in the body.

Recommendations for further research are (1) to determine and compare intake of fluoride from all sources (this recommendation has implications for research design in several of the areas that follow); and (2) to determine the metabolic characteristics of fluoride in infants, young children, and the elderly, as well as in patients with progressive renal disease.

DENTAL FLUOROSIS

Fluoride prevents tooth decay by enhancing the remineralization of enamel that is under attack, as well as inhibiting the production of acid by decay-causing bacteria in dental plaque. Fluoride is also a normal constituent of the enamel itself, incorporated into the crystalline structure of the developing tooth and enhancing its resistance to acid dissolution.

One side effect of too much fluoride ingested in early childhood while teeth are forming, however, is dental fluorosis; the enamel covering of the teeth fails to crystallize properly, leading to defects that range from barely discernible to severe brown stain, surface pitting, and brittleness. Fluoride intake by children 2-5 years old is particularly important because the anterior (front) permanent teeth are at the early-maturation stage, during which they are particularly susceptible to fluoride-induced changes. Dental fluorosis also is a dose-response condition: the greater the fluoride intake during tooth development, the more severe the dental fluorosis. Depending upon the amount and time (relative to tooth development) of fluoride absorbed, severity of dental fluorosis can range from barely discernible to severe manifestations of stained and pitted tooth enamel. PHS's recommended fluoride concentration in drinking water,

0.7-1.2 mg/L, was designed to maximize prevention of dental caries while limiting the prevalence of dental fluorosis to about 10% of the population, virtually all of it mild to very mild. A 1991 report from PHS of the U.S. Department of Health and Human Services compiled the results of independent investigations conducted during the 1980s on dental fluorosis in 24 cities and compared them with a series of PHS surveys conducted during the late 1930s and early 1940s in 21 cities. That comparison showed that the prevalence of dental fluorosis, most of it very mild to mild, had increased. The 1980s data showed that the mean prevalence of dental fluorosis in four cities with optimally fluoridated water supplies was around 22% (17% very mild, 4% mild, 0.8% moderate, and 0.1% severe). In another city with a water fluoride concentration in the range of 1.8-2.2 mg/L, dental fluorosis prevalence was 53% (23% very mild, 17% mild, 8% moderate, and 5% severe). In two other cities with water fluoride concentrations greater than 3.7 mg/L, prevalence was around 84% (25% very mild, 27% mild, 19% moderate, and 14% severe). The data in the PHS report also showed that the greatest relative increase in fluorosis prevalence since the early studies was in communities with very low water fluoride concentrations, demonstrating the influence of sources of fluoride other than water. Those sources make it difficult to estimate fluoride exposure; they represent a source of possible error in estimating fluoride intake in studies of the relation between fluoride exposure and dental fluorosis. Moreover, there is disagreement on whether dental fluorosis (even moderate-to-severe dental fluorosis, in which substantial tooth enamel is affected and dental treatment might be required) is a cosmetic problem or an adverse health effect.

In general, the evidence supports the conclusion that fluoridation at the recommended concentrations, in the absence of fluoride from other sources, results in a prevalence of mild-to-very-mild (cosmetic) dental fluorosis in about 10% of the population and almost no cases of moderate or severe dental fluorosis. At 5 or more times the recommended concentration, the proportion of moderate-to-severe dental fluorosis is substantially higher. The most effective approach to controlling the prevalence and severity of dental fluorosis, without jeopardizing the benefits of fluoride to oral health, is likely to come from more judicious control of fluoride in foods, processed beverages, and dental products, especially those items used by young children.

Recommendations for further research are to identify sources of fluoride during the critical stages of tooth development in childhood and evaluate the contribution of each source to dental fluorosis. Further research should be aimed at the goal of minimizing exposure to fluoride concomitant with maintaining effectiveness in preventing caries.

FLUORIDE AND BONE FRACTURES

The effect of fluoride on bone strength, hip fractures, and skeletal fluorosis in humans has been addressed in two types of studies. The first type involves clinical trials of the effectiveness of high concentrations of fluoride supplements in strengthening bones and preventing further fractures in patients with osteoporosis; this treatment has been used primarily in Europe for almost 30 years. When conducted using proper control groups, these studies showed little or no benefit even at dosages of 20-32 mg per day, well over 10 times the exposure from fluoridated drinking water. If anything, the treated groups experienced a greater number of new fractures, including painful stress fractures in bones other than the vertebrae.

The second type of human study involves epidemiological investigations. These studies compared the rate of bone fracture in populations of the elderly that differed in their exposure to natural or added fluoride in drinking water. Geographic and time-trend analyses were made; time-trend analysis is considered the stronger methodology because there is less opportunity for confounding by other risk factors. Of the six epidemiological studies that used geographic comparisons (where no actual intake data were available), four found a weak association between fluoride in drinking water and the risk of hip fracture. Two additional studies examined time trends in bone fracture before and after water fluoridation: one found no association and the other a negative association. Only two additional studies collected information on individual exposure: one (essentially a geographic comparison) found an increased risk of hip fracture at water fluoride concentrations of 4 mg/L, and the other observed no difference in risk.

Studies with several species of experimental animals have yielded various outcomes. Most of the studies indicated little or no effect on bone strength, even with very high fluoride intake and very high concentrations of fluoride in bone. The subcommittee identified many potential problems in the experimental design of the animal studies, including the lack of suitable control groups with reasonably low fluoride exposures. However, the subcommittee concluded that the weight of evidence indicates that bone strength is not adversely affected in animals that are fed a nutritionally adequate diet unless there is long-term ingestion of fluoride at concentrations of at least 50 mg/L of drinking water or 50 mg/kg in diet.

In view of the conflicting results and limitations of the current data base on fluoride and the risk of hip or other fractures, the subcommittee concludes that there is no basis at this time to recommend that EPA lower the current standard for fluoride in drinking water for this end point. However, the subcommittee recommends additional research to improve the current data base.

A recommendation for further research is to conduct additional studies of hip and other fractures in geographical areas with high and low fluoride concentrations in drinking water and to make use of individual information about water consumption. These studies should also collect individual information on bone fluoride concentrations and intake of fluoride from all sources, as well as reproductive history, past and current hormonal status, intake of dietary and supplemental calcium and other cations, bone density, and other factors that might influence risk of hip fracture.

EFFECTS OF FLUORIDE ON
THE RENAL SYSTEM

Renal excretion is the major route of elimination for inorganic fluoride from the body. As a result, kidney cells are exposed to relatively high fluoride concentrations, making the kidney a potential site for acute fluoride toxicity. Animal studies have shown that very high water fluoride concentrations of 100-380 mg/L can lead to necrosis of proximal and renal tubules, interstitial nephritis, and dilation of renal tubules. However, human epidemiological studies have found no increase in renal disease in populations with long-term exposure to fluoride at concentrations of up to 8 mg/L of drinking water.

The subcommittee concludes that available evidence shows that the threshold dose of fluoride in drinking water for renal toxicity in animals is approximately 50 mg/L. The subcommittee therefore believes that ingestion of fluoride at currently recommended concentrations is not likely to produce kidney toxicity in humans.

EFFECTS OF FLUORIDE ON
THE GASTROINTESTINAL SYSTEM

In the acid environment of the stomach, fluoride and hydrogen ions can combine to form hydrogen fluoride, which, at sufficiently high concentrations, can be irritating to the mucous membranes of the stomach lining. Experimental studies with several animal species have shown dose-dependent adverse effects, such as chronic gastritis and other lesions of the stomach, at fluoride concentrations of 190 mg/L and higher. Reports of gastrointestinal effects in humans often involve workers exposed to unknown concentrations of fluoride in the workplace, so that the contribution of fluoride exposure to the risk of adverse health effects is unknown. The subcommittee noted that these workers could also be exposed to other toxic substances present in the work environment. There have been few studies of the gastrointestinal effects of fluoride at low concentrations.

The subcommittee concludes that the available data show that the concentrations of fluoride found in drinking water in the United States are not likely to produce adverse effects in the gastrointestinal system.

EFFECTS OF FLUORIDE ON
HYPERSENSITIVITY AND THE IMMUNE SYSTEM

Few animal and human data on sodium fluoride-related hypersensitivity reactions are found in the literature. In animal studies, excessively high doses, inappropriate routes of administration of fluoride, or both were used. Thus, the predictive value of those data, in relation to human exposures at accepted exposure levels, is questionable. Reports of hypersensitivity reactions in humans resulting from exposure to sodium fluoride are mostly anecdotal.

The literature pertaining to immunological effects of fluoride is limited. Although direct exposure to high concentrations of sodium fluoride in vitro affects a variety of enzymatic activities, the relevance of the effects in vivo is unclear. Standardized immunotoxicity tests of sodium fluoride at relevant concentrations and routes of administration have not been conducted. The weight of evidence shows that fluoride is unlikely to produce hypersensitivity and other immunological effects.

EFFECTS OF FLUORIDE ON REPRODUCTION

There have been reports of adverse effects on reproductive outcomes associated with high levels of fluoride intake in many animal species. In most of the studies, however, the fluoride concentrations associated with adverse effects were far higher than those encountered in drinking water. The apparent threshold concentration for inducing reproductive effects was 100 mg/L in mice, rats, foxes, and cattle; 100-200 mg/L in minks, owls, and kestrels; and over 500 mg/L in hens.

Based on these findings, the subcommittee concludes that the fluoride concentrations associated with adverse reproductive effects in animals are far higher than those to which human populations are exposed. Consequently, ingestion of fluoride at current concentrations should have no adverse effects on human reproduction.

GENOTOXICITY

Fluoride has been tested extensively for its genotoxicity. It does not damage DNA or induce mutations in microbial systems, but it has produced mutations and chromosomal damage in several in vitro tests with mammalian cells. Sodium fluoride, in particular, inhibits protein and DNA synthesis and has been reported to cause chromosomal aberrations in human cells. The lowest effective dose in these cell-culture studies was a fluoride concentration of approximately 10 μg/mL, whereas the normal concentration in human plasma is 0.02-0.06 μg/mL, even in areas where drinking water is fluoridated, which means that there is a large margin of safety.

Sodium fluoride and other fluoride salts also have been tested for genotoxicity in the fruit fly *Drosophila*, as well as in mice and rats. The subcommittee's review of the results of these in vivo studies was inconclusive, however, because of differences in protocols and insufficient detail to support a thorough analysis. There are no published studies on the genetic or cytogenetic effects of fluoride in humans. The subcommittee concludes that the genotoxicity of fluoride should not be of concern at the concentrations found in the plasma of most people in the United States.

CARCINOGENICITY

More than 50 epidemiological studies have examined the relation between fluoride concentrations in drinking water and human cancer. Most studies compared geographic or temporal patterns of cancer occurrences with distributions of fluoride in drinking water. These studies provide no credible evidence for an association between fluoride in drinking water and the risk of cancer. The existence of such an extensive epidemiological data base on fluoride with no consistent evidence of carcinogenic effects suggests that, if there is any increase in cancer risk due to exposure to fluoride, it is likely to be small. However, most of these studies used geographic and temporal comparisons of cancer rates and hence are of limited sensitivity. Further analytical studies with accurate information on individual fluoride exposures and disease diagnoses are therefore desirable.

The subcommittee also reviewed the literature on the potential carcinogenic effects of fluoride in animals. Although the results of earlier animal studies were largely negative, the studies were not conducted using current bioassay techniques and are thus of limited value. The subcommittee placed greater weight on two recent studies. The first, conducted by the National Toxicology Program (NTP), administered fluoride at concentrations of up to 175 mg/L of drinking water. Although the results were negative for male and female mice and female rats, there was some evidence of a dose-related increase in the incidence of osteosarcomas in male rats. However, these results were not confirmed by a second study conducted by Procter & Gamble, in which fluoride was administered in the diet at doses higher than those in the NTP study. The Procter & Gamble study did produce a significant dose-related increase in the incidence of osteomas (benign bone tumors) in male and female mice. However, these lesions were not considered to be neoplastic and, in any event, have no known counterpart in human pathology. The subcommittee concludes that the available laboratory data are insufficient to demonstrate a carcinogenic effect of fluoride in animals. The subcommittee also concludes that the weight of the evidence from the epidemiological studies completed to date does not support the hypothesis of an association between fluoride exposure and increased cancer risk in humans.

Nonetheless, the subcommittee recommends conducting one or more carefully designed analytical epidemiological (case-control or cohort) studies to more fully evaluate the relation between fluoride exposure and cancer, especially osteosarcomas, at various sites, including bones and joints. In conducting such studies, it is important that individual exposure to fluoride from all sources be determined as accurately as possible.

CONCLUSIONS

Based on its review of available data on the toxicity of fluoride, the subcommittee concludes that EPA's current MCL of 4 mg/L for fluoride in drinking water is appropriate as an interim standard. At that level, a small percentage of the U.S. population will exhibit moderate or even severe dental fluorosis. However, the question of whether to consider dental fluorosis a cosmetic effect or an adverse health effect and the balancing of the health risks and health benefits of fluoride are matters to be determined by regulatory agencies and are beyond the charge or expertise of this subcommittee.

The subcommittee found inconsistencies in the fluoride toxicity data base and gaps in knowledge. Accordingly, it recommends further research in the areas of fluoride intake, dental fluorosis, bone strength and fractures, and carcinogenicity. The subcommittee further recommends that EPA's interim standard of 4 mg/L should be reviewed when results of new research become available and, if necessary, revised accordingly.

Health Effects of
Ingested Fluoride

1 INTRODUCTION

Early in this century, researchers observed that people with dental fluorosis, or mottled teeth, had a lower incidence of dental caries than people without dental fluorosis. Later, naturally occurring fluoride in drinking water was identified as being responsible for the reduction in dental caries. Community studies conducted in the 1940s showed an inverse relation between fluoride in drinking water and dental caries. Those findings led to the public-health practice of adding fluoride to fluoride-deficient water. Since 1962, the "optimal" concentration of fluoride in drinking water for the United States has been set at 0.7-1.2 milligrams per liter (or parts per million),[1] depending on the mean temperature of the locality (0.7 mg/L for areas with warm climates, where water consumption is high, and 1.2 mg/L for cool climates, where water consumption is low). That range has been considered optimal because it provides a balance between prevention of dental caries and occurrence of objectionable dental fluorosis. Objectionable dental fluorosis is a mottling of dental enamel characterized by staining or pitting.

In addition to ingesting fluoride in drinking water, people now receive fluoride from a large number of other sources, such as toothpastes, mouth rinses, soft drinks, tea, processed foods, and vegetables. Fluoride

---

[1]The fluoride level in drinking water can be expressed equivalently as parts per million (ppm) or milligrams per liter (mg/L). Fluoride concentrations in tissues such as bone can be expressed equivalently as parts per million or milligrams per kilogram.

is also added when fluoridated water is used during cooking. Therefore, fluoride intake from sources other than drinking water can be substantial. Despite the apparent success of water fluoridation in reducing the incidence of dental caries, water fluoridation remains controversial. Some people believe that fluoride can cause severe dental fluorosis, which may lead to psychological problems. Assertions have been made that fluoride is related to skeletal fluorosis and subsequent fractures, cancer, soft-tissue effects, and arthritis. Critical analysis of toxicological data on fluoride has shown, however, that important adverse health effects, such as crippling skeletal fluorosis and kidney and other soft-tissue damage, occur in humans only when fluoride concentrations in drinking water exceed 8 mg/L for many years. The controversy escalated in 1975 when those opposed to fluoridation claimed that cancer mortality was higher in areas with fluoridated water than in areas with nonfluoridated water. Although that claim was refuted subsequently by other investigators, the lingering concern over a possible association between fluoridation and cancer prompted the National Toxicology Program (NTP) of the U.S. Department of Health and Human Services to conduct a carcinogenicity bioassay to determine whether sodium fluoride is carcinogenic in mice and rats. The results of the NTP study were published in 1990 in a report entitled "Toxicology and Carcinogenesis Studies of Sodium Fluoride in F344/N Rats and B6C3F$_1$ Mice (Drinking Water Studies)." The results of this study are that

[u]nder the conditions of the 2-year dosed water studies, there was equivocal evidence of carcinogenic activity of sodium fluoride in male F344/N rats, based on the occurrence of a small number of osteosarcomas in dosed animals. 'Equivocal evidence' is a category for uncertain findings defined as studies that are interpreted as showing a marginal increase of neoplasms that may be related to chemical administration. There was no evidence of carcinogenic activity in female F344/N rats receiving sodium fluoride at concentrations of 25, 100, or 175 mg/L sodium fluoride in drinking water for 2 years. There was no evidence of carcinogenic activity of sodium fluoride in male or female mice receiving sodium fluoride at concentrations of 25, 100, or 175 mg/L in drinking water for 2 years.
    Dosed rats had lesions typical of fluorosis of the teeth and female rats receiving drinking water containing 175 mg/L sodium fluoride had increased osteosclerosis of long bones [NTP, 1990].

The NTP findings have further stimulated the controversy regarding the safety of fluoride.

In response to the controversy, especially regarding possible carcinogenicity of fluoride, the U.S. Environmental Protection Agency (EPA) requested that the National Research Council's Board on Environmental Studies and Toxicology (BEST) review the toxicological and exposure data for fluoride and characterize the risk associated with ingested fluoride (e.g., from water and food) and determine whether EPA's current maximum contaminant level (MCL) of 4 mg/L of drinking water is acceptable to protect the public health. In addition, EPA requested identification of gaps in fluoride data and recommendations for future research. In response to EPA's request, this project was assigned to BEST's Committee on Toxicology. The Subcommittee on Health Effects of Ingested Fluoride was established to review the current fluoride toxicity data and drinking-water standards.

This report is the result of a detailed evaluation of possible adverse health effects associated with ingested fluoride. The report examines in detail the current data on carcinogenicity of fluoride in humans and animals, dental fluorosis, skeletal effects, effects on the renal, gastrointestinal, and immune systems, effects on reproduction, and genotoxicity from ingested fluoride. In addition, gaps in knowledge on fluoride toxicity are identified, and recommendations are made to minimize the risk to human health from fluoride ingestion.

Chapter 2 discusses dental fluorosis. Chapter 3 reviews the relation of fluoride intake to bone strength, hip fractures, and skeletal fluorosis. Chapter 4 considers the reproductive toxicity of fluoride. Chapter 5 discusses the effects of fluoride on the renal, gastrointestinal, and immune systems. Chapter 6 reviews the genotoxicity of fluoride. Chapter 7 presents the results of carcinogenicity studies in humans and animals. Chapter 8 considers the pharmacokinetics of fluoride.

2 DENTAL FLUOROSIS

THE FLUORIDE CONTENT OF TEETH

All humans ingest fluoride to some extent, and fluoride's affinity for calcified tissues makes it a normal constituent of dental tissues. Up to 4 times as much fluoride is contained in dentin, the bone-like material that constitutes the bulk of a tooth, as in enamel, the visible outer layer. Fluoride is not evenly distributed in enamel and is concentrated primarily on the outer enamel surface. Most fluoride is incorporated into the crystalline lattice of enamel before tooth eruption, but more is incorporated into the enamel crystals immediately after eruption, while the enamel is still maturing. The capacity for sound, newly erupted teeth to absorb fluoride into the enamel's crystalline lattice, however, rapidly diminishes as the enamel matures (Weatherell et al., 1977). As a result, the amount of fluoride in dental enamel does not increase with age to nearly the same extent as in bone. Enamel that has undergone demineralization, the first histological effect of dental caries, and subsequent remineralization contains higher concentrations of fluoride than does sound enamel (Silverstone, 1977).

The concentration of fluoride in sound, mature tooth enamel, at a depth of approximately 2 micrometers (μm), averages 1,700 ppm in people residing in areas with low concentrations of fluoride in drinking water (i.e., fluoride at 0.1 mg/L or less) and 2,200-3,200 ppm in areas with concentrations of fluoride at approximately 1.0 mg/L. Enamel fluoride concentrations of this order have no adverse impact on oral health; indeed, the presence of fluoride in the crystalline lattice of dental enamel can only increase the enamel's resistance to dissolution in decay-causing acids. When drinking water contains naturally occurring fluoride at 5-7 mg/L (much higher than recommended), enamel fluoride concentrations have been measured at 4,800 ppm (Aasenden, 1974). No data could be found on enamel fluoride concentrations in people residing in areas where drinking water contains 1-5 mg/L. People from areas with high concentrations of naturally occurring fluoride in drinking water (i.e., 5-7 mg/L) usually exhibit severe dental fluorosis, and their enamel can become brittle enough to fracture at incisal edges and cusp tips. Caries might begin in the broken enamel, and, even if it does not, teeth in this condition often require treatment to restore function.

FLUORIDE'S ACTION IN PREVENTING DENTAL CARIES

Various forms of fluoride have been used in American dentistry over the past 40 years to prevent tooth decay. The results have been highly successful, and the prevalence and severity of dental caries in the 1990s are substantially reduced from the levels seen in the 1950s.

Fluoride's action in preventing caries comes from both pre-eruptive and post-eruptive mechanisms (Dawes, 1989). In some studies of water fluoridation, the greatest reductions in caries were seen in children who were born as fluoridation began or thereafter, evidence that supports a pre-eruptive effect (Grainger and Coburn, 1955; Forrest and James, 1965; Horowitz and Heifetz, 1967; Katz and Muhler, 1968; Chandra et al., 1980). However, evidence of caries-preventive effects in teeth already erupted or in the process of erupting when fluoridation began is also long-standing (Klein, 1945, 1946; Arnold et al., 1953; Ast and Chase, 1953; Backer Dirks et al., 1961; Russell and Hamilton, 1961; Backer Dirks, 1967) and has been confirmed more recently (Hardwick et al., 1982). The relative importance of pre-eruptive and post-eruptive effects continues to be researched and debated (Groeneveld et al., 1990;

Horowitz, 1990; Thylstrup, 1990), although the mechanisms of the effects are well-defined.

Pre-eruptively, ingested fluoride is incorporated into the developing enamel hydroxyapatite crystal, where it has the effect of reducing enamel solubility (Beltran and Burt, 1988). Pre-eruptive fluoride might prevent caries more effectively in pit-and-fissure lesions than in smooth-surface caries (Groeneveld et al., 1990).

Post-eruptively, the frequent infusion of low-concentration fluoride into the oral cavity, such as drinking fluoridated water or regular brushing with a fluoride toothpaste, enhances remineralization (i.e., rebuilding of the enamel matrix) when demineralization has occurred in the early stages of the carious process (Koulourides, 1990). Some of the fluoride that comes into the mouth from water, food, or toothpaste concentrates in dental plaque (Singer et al., 1970), where most of it is held in bound rather than free ionic form. The bound fluoride can be released in response to lowered plaque pH that demineralizes enamel (Tatevossian, 1990), and fluoride is taken up more readily by demineralized enamel than by sound enamel (White and Nancollas, 1990). The availability of plaque fluoride to respond to acid challenge leads to gradual establishment of well-crystallized and more acid-resistant apatite in the enamel surface during the frequent demineralization-remineralization cycles (Ericsson, 1977; Thylstrup et al., 1979; Kidd et al., 1980; Chow, 1990; Thylstrup, 1990).

Plaque fluoride also inhibits glycolysis, the process in which sugar is metabolized by bacteria to produce acid. Plaque fluoride can retard the production of extracellular polysaccharide by cariogenic bacteria, a production that is necessary for plaque to adhere to smooth enamel surfaces and, hence, for caries to occur (Hamilton, 1990).

In assessing the relative impact of pre-eruptive and post-eruptive effects of fluoride, it became evident by the mid-1970s that a high concentration of enamel fluoride could not by itself explain the extensive reductions in caries that fluoride produced (Levine, 1976). As described earlier, enamel fluoride concentrations at a depth of 2 μm average 1,700-4,800 ppm, depending on age and fluoride exposure. The theoretical concentration of fluoride in pure fluorapatite that would reduce its acid solubility to the extent necessary to explain all reductions in caries is approximately 38,000 ppm (Wefel et al., 1986). It has also been shown that high concentrations of enamel fluoride do not necessarily mean that caries will not occur (Arends and Christoffersen, 1990). The evidence collectively demonstrates that fluoride prevents caries by post-eruptive actions as well as by pre-eruptive incorporation of hydroxyapatite crystals into the enamel.

In addition, high-concentration fluoride at approximately 12,000 ppm, as used in professionally applied gels, might have a specific bactericidal action on cariogenic bacteria in plaque (Bowden, 1990). Those gels also leave a temporary layer of calcium fluoride on the enamel surface, which is available for release when the pH at the enamel surface is lowered (LeGeros, 1990). The cariogenic bacterium *Streptococcus mutans* has been shown to become less acidogenic through adaptation to an environment where it is regularly exposed to low concentrations of fluoride in drinking water or to higher concentrations in toothpastes and mouth rinses (Rosen et al., 1978; Bowden, 1990; Marquis, 1990). It is plausible, though not confirmed, that this ecological adaptation reduces the cariogenicity of *S. mutans* in humans (van Loveren, 1990).

HISTOPATHOLOGY OF DENTAL FLUOROSIS

Dental fluorosis is a condition of the dental hard tissues; it is not a generalized health effect. It is defined as a hypomineralization of enamel, characterized by greater surface and subsurface porosity than is found in normal enamel, and results from excess fluoride reaching the growing tooth during its developmental stages (Fejerskov et al., 1990). The staining, which is characteristic of more severe forms of fluorosis, actually develops after tooth eruption, but is seen only when porous enamel has formed before eruption (Fejerskov et al., 1990). Surface enamel that exhibits dental fluorosis contains higher concentrations of fluoride than does unaffected enamel, and the fluoride content generally increases with the severity of the condition (Richards et al., 1989). The fluoride content of crystals in the hypomineralized subsurface layer is low, however, when compared with the content of crystals in the more fully mineralized enamel surface layers (Richards et al., 1989; Yanagisawa et al., 1989), and these subsurface crystals appear stunted when examined microscopically.

The process of enamel maturation consists of an increase in mineralization within the developing tooth and a concurrent loss of early-secreted matrix proteins. Excess fluoride available to the enamel during maturation disrupts mineralization and results in excessive retention of enamel proteins. This process has been well-illustrated in animal studies. When rats were given various concentrations of fluoride in their drinking water over a 5-week period, no differences were found in the protein content of fluorotic enamel and control enamel during the secretory phase of enamel formation (Den Besten, 1986). However, in fluorotic enamel during the early-maturation stage, animals receiving high doses of fluoride had more enamel proteins retained. At the late-maturation stage, differences were again less apparent, and only the dental enamel from animals with the highest fluoride intake contained more protein (Den Besten, 1986). This research indicates that the early-maturation stage is the developmental period when enamel is most sensitive to the effects of fluoride.

Other research in various animal models (Richards et al., 1986; Richards, 1990) and humans (Evans and Stamm, 1991a) generally supports the idea that the early-maturation stage is the most critical developmental period for dental fluorosis, but fluoride at sufficiently high concentrations might affect enamel at all stages of its formation (Den Besten and Crenshaw, 1987; Suckling et al., 1988). In humans, the clinical signs of severe dental fluorosis (enamel pitting and obvious brown stain) follow the breakdown of the better-mineralized surface layers of enamel shortly after eruption, resulting in variable uptake of mineral in the exposed hypomineralized subsurface lesions (Thylstrup, 1983; Fejerskov et al., 1991).

Some physiological conditions that affect amelogenesis in humans can lead to variations in the clinical appearance of dental fluorosis at similar levels of fluoride intake (Angmar-Månsson and Whitford, 1990). Calcium deficiency and generalized malnutrition are examples of such conditions seen in many developing countries. Any condition that decreases urinary pH, such as disorders in acid-base balance, can reduce the renal clearance of fluoride and increase the likelihood of dental fluorosis (Whitford and Reynolds, 1979; Ekstrand et al., 1982). Retention of fluoride in body tissues is increased by high altitudes (Manji et al., 1986a), although residing at high altitudes, in the absence of fluoride, has been found to disrupt amelogenesis and produce a condition that can be clinically confused with dental fluorosis (Angmar-Månsson and Whitford, 1990).

Dental fluorosis is a dose-response condition: the greater the intake during developmental periods, the more severe the fluorosis will be (Dean, 1942; Eklund et al., 1987; Larsen et al., 1987; Gedalia and Shapira, 1989; Fejerskov et al., 1990). Evidence from animal studies shows that several patterns of fluoride exposure can disturb amelogenesis. Early research indicated that the development of fluorosis in the continuously growing rat incisor was associated with occasional "spikes" in plasma fluoride concentrations, produced by daily injections, that raised the plasma fluoride concentration above a presumed threshold value (Angmar-Månsson et al., 1976; Myers, 1978). Later research confirmed that finding (Angmar-Månsson and Whitford, 1982) but also showed that relatively constant, slightly elevated concentrations of plasma fluoride produced by constant infusion in rats (approximately 3 micromoles (μmol)/L) also resulted in enamel fluorosis. A subsequent study, which also employed constant infusion of fluoride in rats, extended the dosing period from 1 to 8 weeks. With longer exposure, enamel fluorosis was associated with plasma fluoride concentrations of only 1.5 μmol/L (Angmar-Månsson and Whitford, 1984). Those results were later confirmed by Nelson et al. (1989), who found that more fluorosis-type lesions were produced in sheep after long-term administration of low doses of fluoride than after short-term administration of high doses. Angmar-Månsson and Whitford (1985) also reported that a single high dose of fluoride (0.75 milligram (mg) or more of fluoride per kilogram (kg) of body weight) caused enamel fluorosis in rats, even though the plasma fluoride concentrations returned to pre-dose levels within 24 hours.

It was hypothesized from those results that the pulse loading (single high dose) and subsequent gradual release of fluoride from bone in the vicinity of the developing enamel result in local fluoride concentrations sufficiently high to disturb amelogenesis. That hypothesis was supported by nuclear microprobe analyses, which showed that the enamel and dentin fluoride concentrations were elevated, in a dose-response manner, even 70 days after the single fluoride doses, by which time the rats' incisor teeth would have renewed themselves nearly 2 times (Angmar-Månsson et al., 1990).

Dental fluorosis in humans generally is more severe in teeth that mineralize later in life than in those that mineralize earlier (Larsen et al., 1985, 1987, 1988; Bælum et al., 1987). That finding is usually attributed to greater ingestion of fluoride by older children compared with younger (although, as a function of body weight, there is often little difference in fluoride consumption between older and younger children). Fluorosis is primarily a condition of permanent teeth; the degree of fluorosis reported in primary teeth is generally much less than that found in permanent teeth (Gedalia and Shapira, 1989). Although extensive fluorosis of primary teeth has been reported in areas of the world with high amounts of fluoride ingestion (Thylstrup, 1978; Olsson, 1979; McInnes et al., 1982; Nair and Manji, 1982; Larsen et al., 1985; Mann et al., 1990), it has not been identified as a problem in the United States.

The lower degree of fluorosis in primary teeth was once believed to be due to the placenta acting as a barrier to the passage of fluoride from maternal to fetal blood, but more recent evidence shows that the placenta acts as only a limited barrier to its passage (Gedalia and Shapira, 1989). However, fetal blood concentrations usually are lower than maternal levels. Most fluoride in a tooth's outer enamel layer is deposited during the enamel maturation period before eruption, a developmental phase that lasts only 1-2 years in primary teeth but takes 4-5 years in permanent teeth. The shorter maturation period for primary teeth, added to lower fetal blood fluoride concentrations during their prenatal development, is probably the main reason why fluorosis in primary teeth is unusual outside areas of high-fluoride ingestion.

DIAGNOSTIC ISSUES IN DENTAL FLUOROSIS

Clinical diagnosis of fluorotic lesions has been plagued from the earliest studies by the fact that not all mottling of dental enamel is caused by fluoride. During McKay's initial studies in the early years of this century he referred to this condition as "Colorado brown stain," a comment both on the geographic location of his investigations and on the severity of the condition he found. In his first national publication on the condition (Black and McKay, 1916), however, it was called "mottled enamel." The term mottled enamel has since evolved to cover a range of dental developmental defects, fluorotic and otherwise; whereas the term fluorosis more correctly applies only to dental defects of fluorotic origin. The use of these terms, however, is unfortunately far from uniform.

The diagnostic problems that can arise when measuring the prevalence of dental fluorosis have been well described in the literature (Fejerskov et al., 1988; Cutress and Suckling, 1990). Malnutrition, metabolic disorders, and the presence of other dietary trace elements can lead to diffuse, symmetrical markings on the enamel that closely mimic the appearance of fluorosis. Most cases of dental fluorosis are probably identified correctly by experienced examiners, but high and low population prevalences and individual cases have been reported that are incompatible with the fluoride histories. In such instances, the likelihood of misclassification seems strong. When a fluoride history is taken concurrently with clinical diagnosis, some argue that the information from the history biases the diagnostic process.

Those issues deserve to be addressed seriously. It must be remembered, however, that the risk of misclassification has long been recognized as an inherent problem in epidemiological study of any condition. Standard procedures have been developed to minimize the chances of misclassification in data collection (Lilienfeld and Lilienfeld, 1980) and to reduce its biasing effect in statistical analysis (Kleinbaum et al., 1982). During data collection, misclassification can be minimized by cross-checking with patient records to certify that diagnoses have been classified correctly (Lilienfeld and Lilienfeld, 1980). For dental fluorosis classification, taking a fluoride history seems to be an appropriate part of a difficult diagnosis. Of course, some diagnostic errors will still be made, but probably no more than are made in clinical examinations for caries, loss of periodontal attachment, soft-tissue lesions, or a host of medical conditions.

The alternative approach is to avoid fluorosis misclassification in the data collection by recording less well-defined entities, such as "enamel opacities" or "developmental defects." Whether or not that approach reduces misclassification, it can yield data that are of limited use in answering research questions. For example, it is not easy to interpret the finding that "some type of defective enamel" was found in 50.1% of a group of schoolchildren, and "white diffuse or patchy" opacities were found in 10.2% of them (Dummer et al., 1990). The latter description best fits that of dental fluorosis, but the authors of that report do not use the word fluorosis at all. In another study, "at least one tooth with defective enamel" was found in 63% of children seen, and 4.4% of them showed "diffuse patchy opacities" (Suckling and Pearce, 1984). The latter description is closest to that of dental fluorosis of all the descriptions given in that report, but again the reader is left to make that interpretation. Others compare the proportion of "blemishes" found in people in fluoridated and nonfluoridated areas (Dooland and Wylie, 1989) and the trends in prevalence of "mottling" since the introduction of fluoride toothpastes (Weeks, 1990).

Even though the problem of misclassifying dental fluorosis is recognized during clinical assessments, determination of risk factors for fluorosis seems more likely to be successful when attempts are made to measure the condition directly. Russell's guidelines for distinguishing between enamel opacities of fluoride and nonfluoride origin, now more than 30 years old (Russell, 1961), are still a valid diagnostic guide. Taking a fluoride history, when practical, is also a standard and appropriate epidemiological procedure that should not bias the data collected.

INDEXES FOR DENTAL FLUOROSIS

This section provides a brief description and critique of the most common indexes used to grade dental fluorosis. The detailed clinical criteria and scoring systems for the three most frequently used indexes (Dean's, Thylstrup and Fejerskov's, and the Tooth Surface Index of Fluorosis) are given in Appendix 1.

The first index to grade dental fluorosis was developed by Dean in 1934; he called it the Fluorosis Index, but it is usually referred to as Dean's index. Dean had been assigned by the U.S. Public Health Service to investigate what was then the newly identified condition of dental fluorosis and to determine if it was a public-health problem requiring action. His first index (Dean, 1934) was fairly arbitrary and consisted of a seven-point ordinal scale from normal to severe. After some years of use, Dean modified the index to form the six-point ordinal scale that is still used today (Dean, 1942). The scores from Dean's index are based on the two worst-affected teeth in the mouth and are derived from the whole tooth rather than the worst-affected surface. (Later research by Thylstrup and Fejerskov (1978) states that all surfaces of an affected tooth should be affected equally.) In the examination, teeth are not dried. Dean's index has stood the test of time, but even though it is adequate for broad definition of prevalence and trends, it is not sufficiently sensitive at both ends of the scale for analytical research.

Dean's index inevitably was modified to meet different conditions in different parts of the world. The Thylstrup-Fejerskov (TF) index is an extensive modification of Dean's with a strong biological basis (Thylstrup and Fejerskov, 1978). The 10-point ordinal TF index is more sensitive than Dean's at the high end of the severity scale, and it appears to be more sensitive at the mild end of the scale because its application calls for teeth to be dried, which makes the mildest fluorosis more likely to be detected (Granath et al., 1985; Cleaton-Jones and Hargreaves, 1990). Indeed, the lowest scores in the TF index reflect such mild fluorosis that some have questioned whether those categories should be included in the index as fluorosis categories (O'Mullane and Clarkson, 1990). The TF index has been shown to be a valid indication of fluoride content of fluorotic enamel, although teeth scored in the first three categories of the index had fluoride concentrations that were similar to those in normal enamel (Richards et al., 1989). The TF index might be too sensitive in those categories, which differ only slightly in their clinical appearance, for purposes other than analytical epidemiology (Clarkson, 1989).

The Tooth Surface Index of Fluorosis (TSIF) was developed by researchers at the National Institute of Dental Research in the early 1980s (Horowitz et al., 1984). It is intended to be more sensitive than Dean's index by ascribing a score to each unrestored surface of each tooth (rather than a single tooth score to the two worst-affected teeth in the mouth), by eliminating Dean's category of "questionable," and by providing greater range at the high end of the severity scale. The tooth is not dried during TSIF examination. Whether it achieves greater sensitivity with these means has not been confirmed, although it probably provides a more valid picture of whole-mouth severity than does Dean's index. Its use of staining as a criterion has been criticized (Fejerskov et al., 1990), because staining is a post-eruptive phenomenon that is a function of a person's dietary habits as well as degree of enamel porosity.

The Fluorosis Risk Index (FRI) was developed to relate age-specific fluoride exposure to development of dental fluorosis (Pendrys, 1990). It divides the surfaces of permanent teeth into two developmentally related groups of surface zones, which begin formation either during the first year of life or during the third to sixth years. It was developed specifically for use in case-control studies and thus has clear rules for categorizing subjects as cases, controls, or neither, depending on the distribution of fluorosis found on designated zones of tooth surfaces. The ability of FRI in a case-control study to relate fluorosis to enamel developmental periods permitted identification of risk factors that other indexes could not do (Pendrys and Katz, 1989). Its use is best restricted to analytical epidemiology.

The Developmental Defects of Enamel Index (DDE) was developed by a working group of the Fédération Dentaire Internationale, and, as its name implies, it was intended to be more than a dental fluorosis index (FDI, 1982). One of the reasons given for developing the DDE was that "Classifications based on etiological considerations are premature because only a few defects can be assigned an etiology" (FDI, 1982). The diagnostic problems described in the previous section affect the DDE because it assigns codes for all types of enamel opacities and thus has made it difficult for researchers to classify fluorosis as distinct from other enamel defects. Data analysis in the DDE is also complicated (Clarkson, 1989). A modified version, intended to make identification of fluorosis simpler, has been used in a national survey of Ireland (Clarkson and O'Mullane, 1989). In this survey, diffuse opacities were found to be the discriminating factor between fluoridated and nonfluoridated areas.

All the indexes have strengths and deficiencies, and choice of index should be determined by the purposes of the study. They are not the only systems for classifying dental fluorosis that have been proposed (Al-Alousi et al., 1975; Butler et al., 1985a), but they are the ones most in use at present. The major problem that arises from use of multiple indexes is that direct comparison of prevalence and severity is difficult when classifications of cases of fluorosis vary according to the index used. The review carried out by the U.S. Public Health Service (PHS, 1991) even considered reports in the literature according to the index used, a conservative approach but one that is hard to criticize purely on scientific grounds. In this review, we attempt to pool results but focus comparisons on prevalence and broad categories of "mild to very mild" and "moderate to severe."

DENTAL FLUOROSIS AND FLUORIDE INTAKE

Dean's initial research established 1.0 mg/L as the approximate concentration of fluoride in drinking water that best prevented caries while keeping unsightly dental fluorosis to a minimum (Dean, 1942), but in reaching that conclusion, Dean did not include the likelihood that more water is consumed by people in warm climates than in cool climates. After Dean's work, the "optimal" concentration of fluoride in drinking water for the United States was established by the U.S. Public Health Service to be between 0.7 and 1.2 mg/L, depending on mean temperature of the locality (PHS, 1962). Regions of the country with warm climates (e.g., Arizona and Texas) use 0.7 mg/L as their optimal concentration, and cool regions (e.g., Minnesota and New England) use 1.0-1.2 mg/L. The recommended water fluoride concentrations for ranges of mean temperature in the United States are shown in Table 2-1. The range of 0.7-1.2 mg/L was established after a series of elegant studies in the 1950s that related fluoride concentrations in drinking water to fluorosis prevalence and severity in different climatic regions in the United States (Galagan, 1953; Galagan and Lamson, 1953; Galagan and Vermillion, 1957; Galagan et al., 1957). The results of those studies were confirmed by further research a decade later (Richards et al., 1967). As was the case with all fluoride research at that time, drinking water was virtually the only source of measurable fluoride. (Foods usually contained only trace amounts of fluoride.)

Although fluoride is no longer considered an essential factor for human growth and development (see NRC, 1989), many believe that there is an optimal dose of systemic fluoride for maximal benefit against caries. (This is not the same subject as the "optimal concentration" of fluoride

TABLE 2-1 Water Fluoride Concentrations Recommended for Various Climatic Conditions

Annual Average Maximum Daily Air Temperatures, °F (°C)	Recommended Control Limits, mg/L		
	Lower	Optimum	Upper
50.0-53.7 (10.0-12.0)	0.9	1.2	1.7
53.8-58.3 (12.1-14.6)	0.8	1.1	1.5
58.4-63.8 (14.7-17.7)	0.8	1.0	1.3
63.9-70.6 (17.8-21.4)	0.7	0.9	1.2
70.7-79.2 (21.5-26.2)	0.7	0.8	1.0
79.3-90.5 (26.3-32.5)	0.6	0.7	0.8

Source: PHS, 1962.

in drinking water and should not be confused with it.) But because the controversy regarding pre-eruptive and post-eruptive fluoride action still exists, this issue deserves some scrutiny.

The concept of an optimal dose goes back to the early days of fluoride research in dentistry. In 1943, the normal daily fluoride intake of children 1-12 years old was estimated to be 0.4-1.7 mg, which provided an average intake of fluoride at 0.05 mg/kg of body weight per day (McClure, 1943). Actual fluoride intake for an individual depended on age, diet, and fluoride content of water. That estimate somehow evolved into a recommendation (Farkas and Farkas, 1974) and then to apparent acceptance of 0.05-0.07 mg/kg per day as an optimal dose (Ophaug et al., 1980a).

Despite its dubious genesis, that dose might be a fair estimate, based on empirical evidence, of the upper limit for fluoride intake in children to minimize fluorosis (Burt, 1992). If all fluoride intake comes from drinking water, that dose for a child weighing 10 kg (an average 1-year-old) would be ingested in 0.5-0.7 L of water fluoridated at 1.0 mg/L. For a child weighing 22 kg (an average 6-year-old), it would be ingested in 1.1-1.5 L of water. Because the scientific base is weak, however, the range of 0.05-0.07 mg/kg should not be referred to as an optimal dose, and it should not be considered more than a guide to the upper limit of intake for minimizing fluorosis.

The intake of fluoride that leads to clinically detectable dental fluorosis, relative to body weight at different stages of growth, still requires considerable clarification. Forsman (1977) stated that a daily intake of 0.1 mg/kg was sufficient to cause dental fluorosis, an estimate that was later revised downward to 0.04 mg/kg (Bælum et al., 1987). Studies in Kenya, where naturally occurring high-fluoride drinking water is common in the Rift Valley, led to an even lower estimate of 0.03 mg/kg (Bælum et al., 1987). Other sources of fluoride were not accounted for in those observations, and none of the estimates specified the period of childhood in which the intakes were most critical. The estimates of 0.03-0.04 mg/kg were for those in the lowest categories of the TF index, in which, as noted earlier, the fluoride content of fluorotic lesions is similar to that of normal enamel. Further research is necessary to clarify the relation between fluoride intake in childhood and development of dental fluorosis. Recent estimates of daily intake of fluoride from food and drink by North American children up to 2 years of age are 0.01-0.16 mg/kg in areas without fluoridation and 0.03-0.13 mg/kg in areas with fluoridation (Burt, 1992).

PREVALENCE OF DENTAL FLUOROSIS

Because dental fluorosis is a dose-response condition (Myers, 1983), severity ranges from barely discernible, even to a trained observer, to the most severe manifestations of stained and pitted enamel. Figure 2-1 demonstrates this range, beginning with unaffected enamel in Figure 2-1*A* and ending with severe dental fluorosis in Figure 2-1*F*. The discussion on the prevalence of dental fluorosis, which follows, refers to these grades of severity.

Severe dental fluorosis (Figure 2-1*E* and 2-1*F*) is endemic in parts of the world where extremely high concentrations of fluoride occur naturally in drinking water. In subtropical zones of India, for example, fluoride concentrations as high as 15-16 mg/L have been recorded (Jolly et al., 1968; Chandra et al., 1980; Subbareddy and Tewari, 1985). In addition to severe dental fluorosis, skeletal fluorosis is not uncommon in such areas (Jolly et al., 1968). East Africa and parts of the Middle East also have excessively high concentrations of fluoride in drinking water. In Kenya, fluoride concentrations of over 40 mg/L have been recorded in drinking water; in one study, over 20% of 1,290 boreholes in the Great Rift contained fluoride at more than 5 mg/L (Manji and Kapila, 1986a). As would be expected, severe dental fluorosis is endemic in many parts of those regions (Møller et al., 1970; Olsson, 1979; Walvekar and Qureshi, 1982; Wenzel et al., 1982; Manji et al., 1986b; Manji and Kapila, 1986b; Chibole, 1987; Haimanot et al., 1987; Mann et al., 1987).

FIGURE 2-1 (*Appears on the next two pages*) (*A*) No fluorosis detectable. (*B*) Very mild fluorosis, most noticeable at the tips of the upper and lower incisor teeth; TSIF score 1-2. (*C*) Mild fluorosis. Diffuse white striations visible over much of the upper incisor teeth; TSIF score 3. (*D*) Moderate fluorosis. Some brown stain visible among the white striations on the upper central incisors; TSIF score 4. (*E*) Severe fluorosis. Discrete pitting of the enamel of the upper and lower front teeth; TSIF score 5. More severe confluent pitting can be seen on the lower bicuspid tooth (the lower tooth at the end of the arch); TSIF score 7. (*F*) Severe fluorosis. Discrete pitting and stain visible; TSIF score 6.

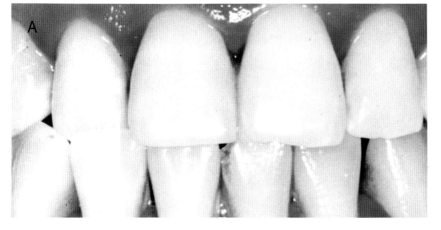

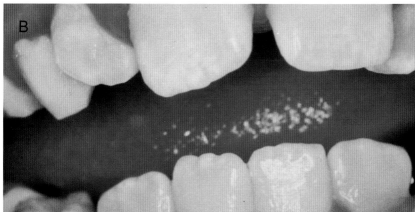

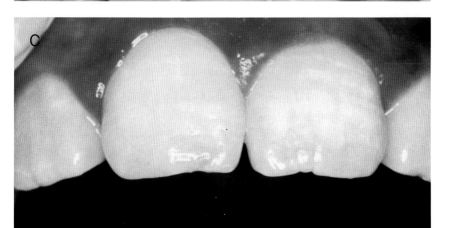

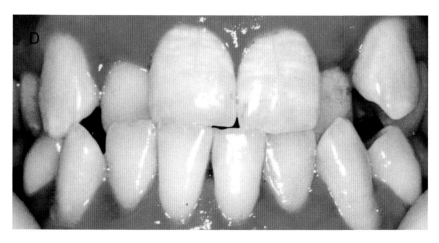

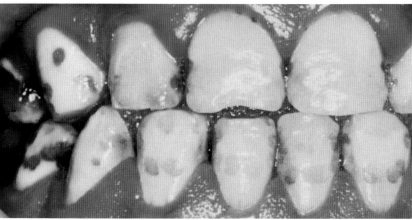

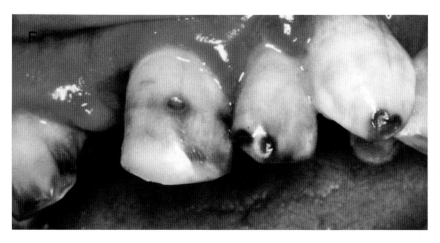

Dean's research during the 1930s and 1940s, conducted in areas with varying amounts of naturally occurring fluoride in drinking water, aimed to establish fluoride concentrations that represented the best balance between low occurrence of caries and acceptable level of dental fluorosis. From his extensive field research, Dean concluded that fluoride at 1.0 mg/L of drinking water was the "minimal threshold of endemic dental fluorosis" and noted that, at 1.0 mg/L, 10-12% of permanent-resident children showed the mildest forms of fluorosis (Figure 2-1*B* and 2-1*C*), mostly in the bicuspids and molars (Dean et al., 1941). Dean's research resulted in acceptance of fluoride at 1.0 mg/L in drinking water as the most appropriate concentration for most of North America, until the climate-related range of 0.7-1.2 mg/L was adopted by the U.S. Public Health Service in 1962. The early supplemental fluoridation studies (fluoride at 1.0 mg/L) in Grand Rapids, Michigan, and Newburgh, New York, conducted at a time when drinking water was virtually the only important source of fluoride, showed that dental fluorosis generally was as prevalent and severe as it was in communities with naturally occurring fluoride at the same concentration (Ast et al., 1956; Russell, 1962).

To establish a "standard" against which the present-day prevalence of dental fluorosis can be assessed, Figure 2-2 shows the distribution of fluorosis in 10 of the many communities studied by Dean in the 1930s and 1940s. The 10 were chosen to demonstrate effects from a range of water fluoride concentrations, and all had more than 50 children of ages 9-14 years in the groups studied. All data were collected by Dean and categorized with Dean's index. Prevalence of fluorosis can be seen to be directly related to fluoride concentration of drinking water up to approximately 4.0 mg/L, after which it tended to level out. Moderate-to-severe dental fluorosis began to be seen at about 1.9 mg/L, and its prevalence rose with increasing fluoride concentrations. It is worth noting that even where drinking water contained fluoride at only 0.4 mg/L, there was some fluorosis recorded, and the relations, although direct, were by no means linear (Dean, 1942).

The research of the 1930s set the stage for controlled addition of fluoride to drinking water at about 1.0 mg/L and was followed by studies through the 1940s and 1950s devoted to evaluating the initial controlled fluoridation projects. After the mid-1960s, however, research into dental fluorosis in the United States dropped off sharply. It was revived only in the 1980s, after Leverett cautioned that fluoride exposure from widespread use of an increasing number of sources of fluoride should be

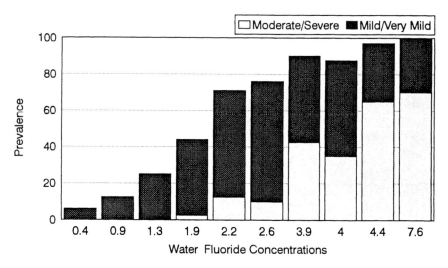

FIGURE 2-2   Prevalence (percent) and severity of dental fluorosis in 10 communities in the United States in the 1930s and 1940s by fluoride concentration (mg/L) in drinking water.   Source: Dean, 1942.

monitored (Leverett, 1982). The new interest in monitoring the impact of fluoride through the 1980s and 1990s yielded evidence that the prevalence of dental fluorosis had increased since Dean's time in both fluoridated and nonfluoridated areas.

In the National Survey of Dental Caries in U.S. School Children in 1986-1987, overall prevalence of dental fluorosis was reported to be 22.3% in children ages 5-17 years (Brunelle, 1989). Nearly all the cases were mild to very mild. Perhaps the most noteworthy aspect of this survey (to date reported only in abstract form) was that prevalence was 18.5% in 17-year-olds and 25.8% in 9-year-olds, a cohort comparison that suggests that childrens' exposure to fluoride increased during the 1970s. (The differing prevalence by age has been suggested to be at least partly due to decreasing fluorosis severity in the same tooth over time, a change attributed to post-eruptive mineralization and to abrasion of affected incisal edges. The issue of whether the milder forms of fluorosis do in fact diminish over time requires further research.) Although dental fluorosis is still more prevalent in fluoridated than in nonfluoridated communities, its prevalence has increased proportionately more in the nonfluoridated areas since Dean's work (Leverett, 1986; Bagramian et al., 1989; Kumar et al., 1989; Williams and Zwemer, 1990).

Several detailed reviews of the literature (Szpunar and Burt, 1987; Pendrys and Stamm, 1990) comparing fluorosis data over time, in addition to other recent research, concluded that the prevalence of dental fluorosis reported in optimally fluoridated areas (both natural and added) in recent years ranged from 8% to 51%, compared with 3% to 26% in nonfluoridated areas. Those ranges consist of all degrees of severity, although 90% or more of fluorosis cases recorded in the United States are in the mild-to-very-mild category. More recently, a prevalence of 80.9% was reported in children 12-14 years old in Augusta, Georgia, the highest prevalence yet reported in an optimally fluoridated community in the United States (Williams and Zwemer, 1990). Again, most of the fluorosis was mild to very mild, but moderate-to-severe fluorosis was found in 14% of the children. Several factors might be contributing to this high prevalence. For example, Augusta is described as optimally fluoridated, but the water fluoride concentrations of 0.9-1.2 mg/L seem excessively high for that climatic region, and over 80% of participants were reported to have used fluoride supplements in childhood (clearly inappropriate in a fluoridated area). Because only 33.4% of eligible children in that study responded to the researchers' initial contact, there is also the possibility of selection bias in the examined group. Pendrys and Stamm (1990) estimated that in the 1930s, residence in an optimally fluoridated area carried about an 18-fold increase in the risk of dental fluorosis, whereas the current increase in risk is about 2-fold. That reduction is largely attributable to an increase in fluorosis in nonfluoridated areas, where fluoride supplements, beverages processed with fluoridated water, and inadvertent swallowing of fluoride toothpaste represent sources of fluoride that were not present in the 1930s.

As can be inferred from the ranges of prevalence already given, the extent of dental fluorosis in a community cannot be estimated from water fluoride concentrations alone. To illustrate, Figure 2-3 shows the prevalence of dental fluorosis in the early 1980s and its distribution, using Dean's index, of categories between mild to very mild and moderate to severe in 16 communities in Texas with varying water fluoride concentrations (reported only as a function of optimal concentration, presumably 0.7 mg/L). The number of examiners in the study was not reported. Although direct comparisons with Dean's data must be made cautiously

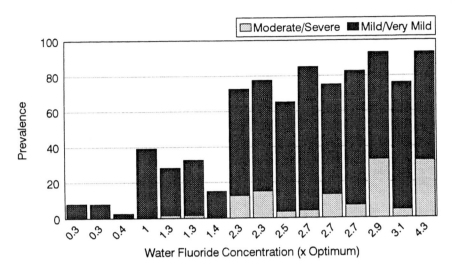

FIGURE 2-3   Prevalence (percent) and severity of dental fluorosis in 16 communities in Texas in the 1980s by fluoride concentration in drinking water. Source: Segreto et al., 1984.

(and there are some curious inconsistencies in the Texas data), prevalence does appear higher in the 1980s than in the 1930s. Prevalence can be seen to vary from 8.7% when water contained 0.3 times the optimal concentration to 94.7% when water contained 4.3 times the optimal concentration (Segreto et al., 1984). The inconsistencies between dental fluorosis prevalence and water fluoride concentrations, seen in Figure 2-3, are difficult to explain. Even though examiner variability is likely to be a factor, the inconsistencies cannot be attributed solely to those variations because the inconsistencies are seen in most series of that kind (e.g., Dean's data in Figure 2-2) and in the ranges of prevalence given in the previous paragraph. They are most likely a result of different individual fluoride intakes, not all of which can be detected without a significant increase in research effort, and variation in individual biological responses to similar fluoride intakes.

Results of semi-longitudinal assessments of dental fluorosis in seven communities in Illinois, conducted by researchers from the National Institute of Dental Research (NIDR), showed the prevalence of fluorosis and its changing distribution in recent years (Heifetz et al., 1988). Those communities were chosen for the varying concentrations of naturally occurring fluoride in their drinking water. Figure 2-4 shows the prevalence and severity of dental fluorosis in children who were 13-15 years old and who were permanent residents in those communities in 1985. Two examiners used the TSIF index, in which grades 1-3 generally correspond to the mildest forms of dental fluorosis and grades 4-7 reflect moderate-to-severe forms. Repeat examinations demonstrated reasonable agreement between the examiners, so their results were pooled. Overall, dental fluorosis prevalence was noticeably higher at the lower fluoride concentrations than Dean had recorded but differed little at 3-4 times the optimal concentration. Moderate-to-severe fluorosis might be even less prevalent, according to these data, than Dean recorded about 50 years earlier.

In their first report, the NIDR researchers concluded that the prevalence of dental fluorosis in children 8-16 years old had not increased significantly since Dean's surveys in the 1930s (Driscoll et al., 1986). That

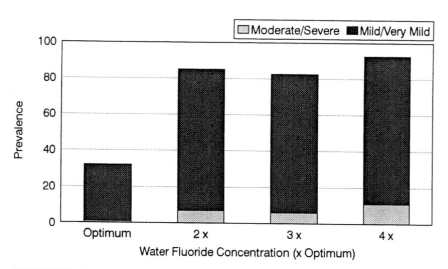

FIGURE 2-4   Prevalence (percent) and severity of dental fluorosis in Illinois in 1985 by fluoride concentration in drinking water. Source: Heifetz et al., 1988.

conclusion was based on data collected in 1980. However, significant increases in prevalence between 1980 and 1985 were reported in cohorts 13-15 years old in the Illinois communities (Heifetz et al., 1988), although they could not be discerned in cohorts 8-10 years old over the same period. Relating age to dental fluorosis and tooth calcification, the authors concluded that fluoride intake (from all sources) had increased from 1970 to 1977 but had not increased much since then.

To focus on the extent of dental fluorosis at higher water fluoride concentrations under modern conditions, Figure 2-5 displays data from three studies in communities where water fluoride concentrations were twice the optimal concentration or higher. Overall, prevalence is high, and most variation seems to come from the proportion of dental fluorosis graded moderate to severe or mild to very mild. It is difficult to specify how much of the variation is due to differences among examiners, varying intakes of fluoride in water and in other sources, differences in other aspects of diet or physiology, individual biological variations, or some combination of those possibilities.

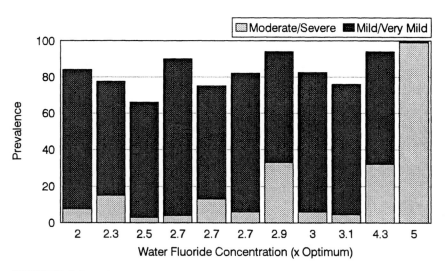

FIGURE 2-5   Prevalence (percent) and severity of dental fluorosis since 1980 for selected communities in the United States with above-recommended fluoride concentrations in drinking water. Sources: Segreto et al., 1984; Eklund et al., 1987; Heifetz et al., 1988.

A 1991 report from PHS compiled the results of independent investigations conducted during the 1980s on dental fluorosis in 24 cities and compared them with a series of PHS surveys conducted during the late 1930s and early 1940s in 21 cities (Table 2-2). That comparison showed that the prevalence of dental fluorosis, most of it mild to very mild, had increased, although the modern-day effects of fluoride from sources other than water were not controlled for. The 1980s data showed that the mean prevalence of dental fluorosis in four cities with optimally fluoridated water supplies was about 22% (17% very mild, 4% mild, 0.8% moderate, and 0.1% severe). In another city with a water fluoride concentration in the range of 1.8-2.2 mg/L, dental fluorosis prevalence was 53% (23% very mild, 17% mild, 8% moderate, and 5% severe). In two other cities with water fluoride concentrations greater than 3.7 mg/L, prevalence was about 84% (25% very mild, 27% mild, 19% moderate, and 14% severe). The data in the PHS report also showed that the greatest relative increase in fluorosis prevalence since the early studies was in communities with very low water fluoride concentrations, demonstrating the influence of sources of fluoride other than water. Those sources make it difficult to estimate fluoride exposure; they represent a confounding factor in studies of the relation between fluoride exposure and dental fluorosis.

RISK FACTORS IN DENTAL FLUOROSIS

Dental fluorosis is a function of total fluoride intake during critical dental developmental periods, and in modern conditions, fluoride is ingested from numerous sources in addition to drinking water. Research efforts to measure the quantities ingested from all such sources are often frustratingly imprecise, because quantifying fluoride intake from current and past use of water, food, and toothpaste, together with past intake from supplements or infant formula, can be extremely difficult. No tissues of the body can be measured for lifetime intake of fluoride. Measurements in plasma might be the best but can be affected by changes in recent intake. As a relatively invasive procedure, it is also not easy to use in field studies. Bone obviously cannot be biopsied from volunteer study participants. Nail clippings reflect only fairly recent fluoride intake and can be readily contaminated.

Despite these measurement problems, risk factors for dental fluorosis

TABLE 2-2 Percent Prevalence of Dental Fluorosis by Clinical Classification and Concentration of Water Fluoride from Dean's 1940 21-City Survey and 1980's Survey Using Dean's Index

Water Fluoride, mg/L	Total No. Cities and Studies		Mean Sample Size per City and Study		Prevalence, %[a] Very Mild	
	1940s	1980s	1940s	1980s	1940s	1980s
<0.4	10	5	360	326	0.9 ± 0.7	4.4 ± 3.0
0.4-0.6	3	1	427	126	5.0 ± 1.4	2.4
0.7-1.2	4	4	270	471	12.3 ± 2.3	17.7 ± 16
1.3-1.7	1	3	477	175	27.0 ± 4.2	19.5 ± 4.1
1.8-2.2	2	1	222	143	35.1 ± 7	23.1
2.3-2.7	1	5	404	174	42.1	40.5 ± 7
2.8-3.2	0	3		124		26.2 ± 16
3.3-3.7	0	0				
>3.7	0	2		163		24.8 ± 11
Total	21	24				

[a]Mean ± standard deviation.
Note: The 21 cities represented in the 1940s column are those cities surveyed by Dean in the 1940s. The 24 cities represented in the 1980s column are those cities surveyed by different investigators using Dean's index in the 1980s. The means and standard deviations are derived from the cities classified by respective water fluoride concentrations.
Source: PHS, 1991.

have been identified from epidemiological study, but it is still difficult to rank their importance with any certainty. One such risk factor is obviously a high fluoride concentration in drinking water (Szpunar and Burt, 1988); even minor adjustments in water fluoride concentrations can lead to significant changes in the prevalence of clinically detectable fluorosis (Evans and Stamm, 1991b). Other risk factors are ingestion of

Prevalence, %ª (Continued)

Mild		Moderate		Severe		Total	
1940s	1980s	1940s	1980s	1940s	1980s	1940s	1980s
0	2.2 ± 2.8	0	0.1 ± 0.3	0	0	0.9 ± 0.7	6.4 ± 2.6
0.6 ± 0.3	0	0	0	0	0	5.6 ± 1.2	2.4
1.4 ± 0.4	4.4 ± 2.0	0	0.8 ± 0.3	0	0.1 ± 0.3	13.6 ± 2.0	22.2 ± 14
3.1 ± 1.1	5.6 ± 4.7	0	0.7 ± 0.6	0	0	30.2 ± 4.3	25.7 ± 9
7.5 ± 2	16.8	1.1 ± 0.1	8.4	0	4.9	44.0 ± 6	53.2
21.3	29.5 ± 5	8.9	8.4 ± 5	1.5	0	73.8	78.5 ± 9
	30.0 ± 11		15.0 ± 16		2.8 ± 5		74.0 ± 22
	27.8 ± 4		19.3 ± 17		13.9 ± 12		83.4 ± 16

fluoride (both intentional and inadvertent) from sources other than drinking water. Indeed, most dental researchers (Horowitz, 1991; Rozier, 1991; Szpunar and Burt, 1992) believe that the best approach to stabilizing the prevalence and severity of dental fluorosis is to control fluoride ingestion from foods, processed beverages, and dental products rather than reduce the recommended concentrations of fluoride in drinking water.

A large number of studies have concluded that fluoride supplements are a risk factor for dental fluorosis (Holm and Andersson, 1982; Suckling and Pearce, 1984; Hellwig and Klimek, 1985; Bohaty et al., 1989; Dooland and Wylie, 1989; Kumar et al., 1989; Larsen et al., 1989;

Pendrys and Katz, 1989; Woolfolk et al., 1989; Wöltgens et al., 1989; Holt et al., 1990; Ismail et al., 1990; Riordan and Banks, 1991; Lalumandier, 1992); however, the relation shown was weak in some of the reports. Other studies have failed to show such a relation (Butler et al., 1985b; Bagramian et al., 1989; Stephen et al., 1991). Fluoride supplements are used widely (Brunelle and Carlos, 1990) and often are prescribed inappropriately (Pendrys and Morse, 1990; Levy and Muchow, 1992). Some of the compliance data are imprecise, however, because use is usually documented retrospectively. It is not clear whether it is solely the misuse of supplements that results in dental fluorosis or whether use at recommended dosages produces the condition (Workshop Report, 1992). In either case, the appropriateness of the recommended supplementation schedules should be considered.

The swallowing reflex is not fully developed in children of preschool age, and their inadvertent swallowing of fluoride toothpaste has been identified as a risk factor (Hellwig and Klimek, 1985; Osuji et al., 1988; Pendrys and Katz, 1989; Milsom and Mitropoulos, 1990; Lalumandier, 1992). However, the fluorosis reported was often very mild and barely discernible. In addition to toothpaste, prolonged use of infant formula in the fluoridated area of Toronto, Ontario, was identified as a risk factor for dental fluorosis (Osuji et al., 1988). High socioeconomic status also emerged as a strong risk factor in a well-conducted case-control study (Pendrys and Katz, 1989), but that finding has not been confirmed in other studies (Bagramian et al., 1989; Hamdan and Rock, 1991). Fluoride in foods and beverages processed with fluoridated water has long been suspected as a risk factor but has not been clearly demonstrated. Unexpectedly high fluoride concentrations in particular foods and beverages (Clovis and Hargreaves, 1988; Burt, 1992; Pang et al., 1992), however, might stimulate further research in this area.

Although the subject has received little attention, some data suggest that dental fluorosis is more prevalent among African-Americans than among other races or ethnic groups in the same community. Russell (1962), in the Grand Rapids fluoridation study, noted that fluorosis was twice as prevalent among African-American children than white children. In the Texas surveys in the 1980s, the odds ratio for African-American children having dental fluorosis, compared with Hispanic and non-Hispanic white children, was 2.3 (Butler et al., 1985b). Dental fluorosis also tended to be more severe among African-American children than white children in the Georgia study (Williams and Zwemer, 1990), although the difference was not statistically significant. In Kenya, prevalence and number of severe cases were unexpectedly high when related to fluoride concentrations in drinking water (Manji et al., 1986c), although nutritional factors could have confounded these results. The reasons for these findings are unknown and do not appear to have been explored further.

THE RELATION BETWEEN DENTAL FLUOROSIS AND CARIES

Dean's studies of this relation in the 1930s showed a sharp reduction in caries prevalence when communities were ranked from the lowest water fluoride concentrations (virtually zero) to approximately 1.0 mg/L. His data also indicated that caries prevalence leveled out when communities with water fluoride concentrations above 1.0 mg/L were rank-ordered (Dean, 1942). On the other hand, caries prevalence was observed to increase when fluoride concentrations were such that severe dental fluorosis was common and the enamel of affected individuals was friable and liable to fracture (Grobler et al., 1986). Other data on the relation are inconsistent. Some studies have found that data follow the J-shaped path shown in Figure 2-6: with increasing fluoride concentrations, caries prevalence diminishes to a certain point and then increases again. However, a different relation is seen in Figure 2-7, in which caries experience among adults in Lordsburg, New Mexico, which had 5 times the optimal fluoride concentration in drinking water, was below that found in the neighboring community of Deming, which had an optimal concentration. Differences were found in the amount of dental treatment received between the two communities, however, a factor that could have influenced the results. An earlier Texas study also reported that caries prevalence among children 12-15 years old continued to diminish even when community fluoride concentrations were 6-8 times the optimal concentration (Englander and DePaola, 1979). These contradictory findings are difficult to explain and merit further research.

CONCLUSIONS

The data show that the prevalence of dental fluorosis, nearly all of it

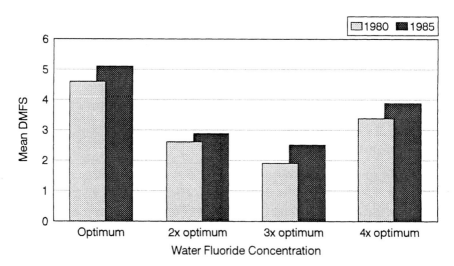

FIGURE 2-6   Caries experience of children 13-15 years of age in Illinois in 1980 and 1985 relative to the fluoride concentration in community drinking water. DMFS = decayed, missing, and filled surfaces. Source: Heifetz et al., 1988.

mild to very mild (Figure 2-1B and 2-1C), rises with increasing fluoride concentrations in drinking water. The data also show fairly consistently that a small, though measurable, proportion of a population exhibits moderate-to-severe dental fluorosis with 1.8-2.0 times the optimal concentration of fluoride in drinking water, and this proportion generally increases with increasing concentrations of fluoride. However, the data are not consistent enough to permit a firm definition of the relation between moderate-to-severe dental fluorosis and water fluoride concentrations. In addition, other uses of fluoride, independent of water fluoride concentrations, clearly affect the prevalence of dental fluorosis. Development of a firm public-policy recommendation is also inhibited by lack of knowledge of the public's perception of less-than-severe fluorosis (Figure 2-1B, 2-1C, and 2-1D).

Public policy on use of fluoride to promote oral health should be aimed at keeping dental fluorosis prevalence as low as possible relative to the benefits of caries control, a classic public-health trade-off. When

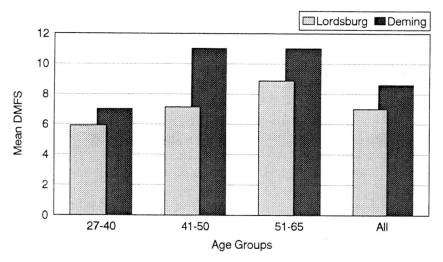

FIGURE 2-7   Caries experience of adults 27-65 years of age in Deming (fluoride at 0.7 mg/L) and Lordsburg (fluoride at 3.5 mg/L), New Mexico, in 1984. Source: Eklund et al., 1987.

drinking water is the only source of fluoride, the evidence supports the conclusion that water fluoridation at currently recommended concentrations results in prevalence of mild-to-very-mild dental fluorosis of about 10% and very little severe fluorosis. At twice the recommended concentrations, the prevalence of moderate-to-severe dental fluorosis is small but measurable. At higher concentrations in drinking water, the prevalence increases, although limited evidence shows that the extent and distribution of dental fluorosis at 4 times the optimal concentration is not much higher than that at 2 times the optimum. At 5 times or more, however, the prevalence of moderate-to-severe dental fluorosis is substantially higher.

Interpretation of current data is difficult because of exposure to fluoride from sources other than drinking water. In the modern U.S. environment, people are exposed to fluoride from food, beverages, toothpaste, and a variety of prescribed or over-the-counter dental products. Many of these are intended for topical use only, but some inadvertent ingestion, especially by young children, is unavoidable. The most effective approach to stabilizing the prevalence and severity of dental fluorosis, without jeopardizing the benefits to oral health, is likely to come from more judicious control of fluoride in foods, processed beverages, and dental products, rather than a reduction in the recommended concentrations of fluoride in drinking water. But applying such a policy would be formidable; reduction of fluoride concentrations in drinking water would be easier to administer, monitor, and evaluate. If it proved to be scientifically justified, such a policy could be considered.

Current regulations of EPA are that the maximum contaminant level (MCL) for fluoride in drinking water is 4.0 mg/L, regardless of mean temperature. That standard is considered low enough to prevent crippling skeletal fluorosis, and dental fluorosis is accepted as a purely cosmetic defect with no general health ramifications. However, the most severe forms of dental fluorosis might be more than a cosmetic defect if enough fluorotic enamel is fractured and lost to cause pain, adversely affect food choices, compromise chewing efficiency, and require complex dental treatment. Severe dental fluorosis has been seen in the United States at 3.5 mg/L (in a warm climate, 5 times the recommended fluoride concentration), but even in that community the ramifications of fluorosis were insufficient to recommend a reduction in the MCL. This conclusion points out the need to revise the PHS guidelines related to temperature and for more information on the impact on general health that results from damage to teeth as a consequence of the severest forms of fluorosis. If recommended fluoride concentrations in drinking water should still be expressed in a range related to mean temperature, the MCL might also be expressed more logically as a temperature-related range rather than a single figure.

Overall, the evidence of the current current relation of dental fluorosis to fluoride in drinking water in the United States is still sparse, and the evidence that does exist is too inconsistent to be used as a basis for recommending changes in EPA regulations. When the results of further research become available, EPA's regulations might need further review and modification.

RESEARCH RECOMMENDATIONS

Studies should be conducted on the sources of fluoride during the critical stages of tooth development in children and on the contribution of the various sources to dental fluorosis etiology. Such information would permit more precise regulation of fluoride products to control fluorosis while retaining fluoride's substantial cariostatic benefits. Studies should be conducted on the relation between water fluoride concentrations and dental fluorosis in various climatic zones. Findings could serve as a basis for any needed revision of the 1962 PHS guidelines. The lowest concentration of fluoride in toothpaste that produces acceptable cariostasis should be determined. That information would permit the marketing of children's toothpastes that would retain anticaries benefits while minimizing the risk of fluorosis.

Further studies should be conducted on the contribution of ingested fluoride and fluoride applied topically to teeth to prevent caries. The results would permit more efficient use of fluoride for caries prevention, thus reducing the risk of fluorosis.

3 FLUORIDE EXPOSURE AND RISK OF BONE FRACTURE

BONE FRACTURE IN HUMANS

Information from two types of studies on bone fracture and case reports of skeletal fluorosis address a possible link between fluoride and bone fracture. One group of studies involved clinical trials designed to test the efficacy of fluoride supplements in strengthening bone and preventing further fractures in those with osteoporosis. Physicians have used fluoride for those purposes for almost 30 years, but until recently, there were no data from systematic, well-controlled clinical trials that addressed the question. Typically, exposure to sodium fluoride in these studies ranged from 50 to 80 mg per day, more than an order of magnitude above the typical exposure to fluoride from fluoridated drinking water. A second group of studies analyzed bone-fracture rates among persons exposed to fluoridated and to nonfluoridated drinking water. With two exceptions, these studies used population data and an ecological design. (Studies of geographic or temporal association, in which population rather than individual data are used, are called ecological studies.) The limitations of this type of study are well known and are described later. Some of the information reviewed here was presented at a workshop on fluoride, hip fractures, and bone health held at the National Institutes of Health (Gordon and Corbin, 1992).

Clinical Trials of Fluoride

Four recent clinical trials with random, controlled designs provide information on exposure to relatively high concentrations of fluoride among high-risk groups for fractures related to osteoporosis. The daily intake of the human subjects in these trials ranged from 50 to 80 mg of sodium fluoride (about 40% fluoride, or 20-32 mg) per day. These fluoride intakes are approximately 10-15 times those of people in the highest decile of drinking-water consumption who live in areas where water is fluoridated at 1 mg/L.

Dambacher et al. (1986) conducted a clinical trial of 15 osteoporotic patients treated with sodium fluoride at 80 mg per day and 14 placebo-treated controls. In the first year, the fracture rate of treated patients was significantly higher than that of the untreated group, but no differences were observed in the second and third years of the trial. After 3 years, the cancellous bone density of treated patients was 8% higher than untreated patients, but total bone density was not increased. Forty-seven percent of the treated group experienced osteoarticular pain and swelling in the lower extremities, attributed to stress fractures, whereas no untreated osteoporotic patients experienced these symptoms. Gastric distress was not observed. Based on results of previous studies by the authors, neither calcium nor vitamin D was added during the trial.

Mamelle et al. (1988) conducted a randomized trial of osteoporotic patients in France with at least one nontraumatic vertebral crush fracture. Treatment with 50 mg of sodium fluoride per day, supplemented with 1 g calcium and 800 international units of vitamin D, was administered to 257 patients, and 209 patients received other standard treatment regimens that did not include sodium fluoride. The number of vertebral crush fractures in the first year was similar in the two groups, and the mean number was significantly lower in the sodium-fluoride-treated patients in the second year. Ankle and foot pain was elevated in the treated group and digestive disorders occurred with equal frequency in the sodium fluoride and other treatment groups.

Two double-blind, placebo-controlled trials were supported by the National Institute of Arthritis and Musculoskeletal and Skin Diseases and conducted at the Mayo Clinic (Riggs et al., 1990) and the Henry Ford Hospital (Kleerekoper et al., 1989). Sodium fluoride was administered at 75 mg per day in both trials, and patients received 500 mg of calcium daily in addition to sodium fluoride or placebos.

Riggs et al. (1990) reported data from a 4-year trial of 202 randomized patients with osteoporosis and vertebral fractures. Sixty-six women in the fluoride group and 69 women in the placebo control group completed the trial. Among those receiving fluoride, bone-mineral density, as measured by dual-photon absorptiometry, increased by 35% ($p <$ 0.0001) in the lumbar spine (mostly trabecular bone) and 12% in the femoral neck ($p < 0.0001$) but decreased by 4% ($p < 0.02$) in the radius (predominantly cortical bone). The number of new vertebral fractures was slightly lower in the sodium-fluoride treatment group, but the number of nonvertebral fractures was significantly higher in the treatment group ($p < 0.01$) than in the control group. The relative risk for nonvertebral fractures, either incomplete or complete fractures, was 3.2 (95% confidence interval (CI) = 1.8-5.6); 61 patients treated with sodium fluoride had 72 nonvertebral fractures, and 24 controls had 24 fractures, either complete or incomplete. There were six hip fractures in the sodium-fluoride treatment group (three incomplete and three complete), and one (complete) hip fracture in the control group. Fifty-four women treated with sodium fluoride and 24 controls experienced side effects, mostly gastrointestinal symptoms and lower-extremity pain, warranting dose reduction.

In the Henry Ford Hospital study, Kleerekoper et al (1989) found no significant difference in vertebral fractures between the sodium fluoride and the control groups. As in the Mayo Clinic study, gastrointestinal side effects and episodes of lower-extremity pain were much more common in the sodium-fluoride group than in the control group. On bone biopsy, 17% of those treated with sodium fluoride had mineralization defects, whereas none was present in the controls.

Population Studies

The risk of bone fracture in the elderly has been studied in populations exposed to naturally occurring or added fluoride in drinking water and compared with groups exposed to low concentrations of fluoride in drinking water. Of the 10 studies considered by the subcommittee, two of the investigations used information from individuals and eight relied on population-based statistics collected for other purposes.

Studies Using Information from Individuals

Cauley et al. (1991) recently reported on data from participants of an ongoing study of osteoporotic fractures in women in the Pittsburgh area. Residential histories and drinking-water sources were gathered from 1950 to 1990 for 1,878 white women ranging in age from 65 to 93 years (mean = 70.9 years). About 10% of the women had exposures to fluoride in drinking water of 1 mg/L for more than 20 years, and 58% had negligible exposures. Public water constituted 73% of exposure-years, and the mean duration of exposure was 6.0 ± 9.24 years (range 0-38 years). No association was found between years of fluoride exposure and bone mineral density with or without adjustment for body-mass index and age. There was also no association with history of fracture. The authors concluded that "these data do not support a protective relation between exposure to fluoridated water and bone mineral density in this population of elderly women."

Women in three small communities in northwest Iowa, who had resided in the same town for at least 5 years, were the subjects in a study by Sowers et al. (1991). The communities were ethnically similar and all eligible women were of Northern European background. One community had water with natural fluoride at high concentrations (4 mg/L), a second had unusually high calcium concentrations, and the third, used as a comparison community, had fluoridated water (1 mg/L) and normal calcium concentrations. Here, we restrict our attention to the comparison between the two communities with high and normal fluoride concentrations. There were 417 subjects in the high-fluoride-concentration community and 194 in the comparison area; they were first enrolled in 1983-1984 and contacted for followup 5 years later; overall participation rates were 74% and 63%, respectively, at followup.

Significantly lower radial bone mass was observed in both younger and older women in the high-fluoride-concentration community. Bone density of the proximal femur was clinically similar in women in the two communities. Postmenopausal, but not premenopausal, women in the high-fluoride community reported significantly more fractures. Relative risk estimates of fracture were adjusted for body-mass index, age, and thiazide use. The 5-year relative risk for any fracture among menopausal women was 2.1 (CI = 1.02-4.4) and for wrist, spine, or hip fractures, 2.2 (CI = 1.1-4.7). The 5-year fracture rate among premenopausal women was also elevated in the high-fluoride community, but chance could not be excluded (relative risk = 1.8, CI = 0.45-8.2). This study from Iowa is discussed here because extensive information on water consumption, use of replacement estrogens, and other factors was gathered from individual participants. However, little of the data from individuals has been reported, and the analyses were essentially ecological in character.

Studies Using Population Characteristics

Eight studies have examined the geographic correlation between hip fracture rates and consumption of fluoridated water or changes in hip fracture rates in the same geographic area before and after fluoridation was begun. The ability of ecological studies to detect excess risk is limited in several respects: (1) lack of individual information on specific exposures, including fluid ingestion patterns and exposure to fluoride from sources other than drinking water, of affected and unaffected members of the population; (2) inability to measure fluoride exposures of study subjects who migrated into study areas before diagnosis of disease or death; and (3) limited or nonexistent possibility of adjusting for differences in risk (confounding) factors, such as smoking, occupational exposures, exogenous estrogens, and dietary patterns, that might influence differences in disease rates in fluoridated and nonfluoridated areas. Confounding can give rise to spurious results, such as positive associations that are not truly present, or alternatively, positive associations that are masked. To the extent that migration is a factor, it is likely to diminish the sensitivity of a geographic correlation study to detect excess risk. An additional problem can arise in correlational studies that use mortality statistics, as occurs in many of the studies of fluoride and cancer, because geographic variation in mortality might reflect differences in access to, or quality of, medical care, and not differences in underlying disease incidence. In this regard, it is helpful to distinguish between ecological studies that make geographically based comparisons and those with a time-trend design. The latter are less subject to confounding from many factors, because they use rates from the same geographic area. Consequently, time-trend studies are considered to have the stronger design. In some cases, ecological studies that show positive associations might be more likely to be published or more rapidly published than those that show no associations. When such publication bias exists, literature is likely to be biased toward showing positive effects. The phenomenon of publication bias is less likely to occur with results from case-control or retrospective-cohort studies, because the large effort involved in conducting these studies is usually attended by an early commitment to publish, regardless of outcome. Given the limitations of ecological studies, most epidemiologists consider them valuable in indicating the likelihood of positive links or in demonstrating the feasibility of hypotheses. When results from a number of such studies (conducted in different times and places) converge to indicate either an exposure-disease relation or no such relation, confidence in the collective findings is bolstered. When many studies fail to observe exposure-disease relations, the possibility of small risks or protective effects, undetected at a population level, cannot be excluded.

In a report presented at a workshop on drinking-water-fluoride influence on hip fracture and bone health held at the National Institutes of Health (see Gordon and Corbin, 1992), Keller (1991) compared hip fracture rates in 216 U.S. counties with natural fluoride concentrations greater than 0.7 mg/L and with rates in 95 counties with naturally low fluoride concentrations (less than 0.4 mg/L) in drinking water. The counties with high concentrations were placed in four groups (0.7-1.2, 1.3-2.0, 2.1-3.9, and 4.0 mg/L and above). Hip fracture ratios were calculated as the reported fracture rate in these county groups divided by the rate in counties with low fluoride concentrations. At optimal fluoride concentrations (0.7-1.2 mg/L), no significant increase in hip fracture ratio was found (risk ratio = 1.016). However, Keller found significant increases in hip fracture ratio at higher concentrations of fluoride in drinking water. The adjusted risk ratio was 1.224 for counties in the highest exposure group. In addition to the usual limitations of ecological studies, this investigation was limited by lack of control for other demographic factors in the computations.

In another study presented at the workshop, May and Wilson (1991) used data from 438 U.S. counties with populations greater than 100,000, representing 70% of the U.S. population. The percentage of the population that received natural or added fluoride in drinking water (approximately 1 mg/L) was estimated for each county. As the percentage of persons exposed to fluoride in water increased, the hip fracture rate generally increased. The regression coefficients (R) were calculated as change in hip fractures per 1,000 persons at risk for each 1% of the population receiving fluoridated water at a concentration of approximately 1 mg/L. The value was significant for white men (R = 0.0037, CI = 0.002-0.005) but not significant for white women (R = 0.0016, CI = 0.001-0.005). In an additional analysis using data from 51 counties (more than 80% of the population was exposed to fluoride), including data on duration of exposure to fluoridated water, the hip fracture rate was higher in counties with up to 10 years of exposure, about 20% lower in counties with 11-18 years of exposure, and intermediate in counties with more than 18 years of exposure. As in the Keller study, this study was limited by the lack in regression models of county demographic factors other than fluoridation status.

Jacobsen et al. (1990) examined hip fracture risk among white women in more than 3,000 counties throughout the United States. Weighted least-squares regression methods were used to examine the association of age-adjusted county hip fracture incidence rates in each county with the percentage of the county population exposed to natural or added fluoride in drinking water. The data were weighted by the number of white women over the age of 65 years. After adjustment for other study variables (i.e., poverty rate, percentage of land in farms, water hardness, sunlight, and latitude), the regression coefficient was statistically significant (R = 0.003, p = 0.0009). It should be noted that weighting of regression equations directly by population size might place too much emphasis on counties with large populations. It is often more appropriate to weight least-squares regression equations by the square root of the population, proportional to the standard error of the estimate.

In another geographic comparison study, Jacobsen et al. (1992) examined hip fracture rates in 129 fluoridated and 194 nonfluoridated counties that had been the subject of a National Cancer Institute study of cancer mortality and fluoridation. More than half of the eligible counties were urban and had natural fluoride concentrations of less than 0.3 mg/L. The proportion of the population receiving fluoridated water in fluoridated counties increased from less than 10% to more than 67% within a

3-year period. Nonfluoridated counties had less than 10% of the population receiving fluoridated water. A small but significant positive association was found between fluoridated water and hip fracture among white men (relative risk = 1.17, CI = 1.1-1.2) and white women (relative risk = 1.1, CI = 1.06-1.10) over 65 years of age. The counties most recently (0-5 years) fluoridated had the highest rates of hip fracture; rates were lower in counties with longer fluoridation exposure.

Jacobsen et al. (1993) also examined hip fracture rates in Rochester, Minnesota, for the 10-year period before and the 10-year period after the drinking-water supply was fluoridated in 1960. The overall annual incidence among persons 50 years of age and older was 483 (CI = 370-597) per 100,000 in 1950-1959, and 450 (CI = 362-537) per 100,000 in 1960-1969. Using Poisson regression models to control for calendar time and age, they found that the relative risk associated with fluoridation was 0.60 (CI = 0.46-0.86) for women and 0.78 (CI = 0.37-1.66) for men.

In another time-trend study, Goggin et al. (1965) compared femoral fracture rates in Elmira, New York (1960 population 46,517) during the 5 years before and the 5 years after fluoridation of the city's water supply in 1959. Femoral fracture rates for Elmira women 60 years of age or older did not differ significantly before or after fluoridation occurred.

In a geographic comparison study from Utah, Danielson et al. (1992) compared the incidence of femoral neck fractures in patients over 65 years of age living in a fluoridated community with the incidence in two nonfluoridated areas. The outcome measure was the rate of hospital discharge for hip fracture. Among women, the age-adjusted risk ratio was 1.27 (CI = 1.08-1.46) and among men, 1.41 (CI = 1.00-1.81). These ratios were based on hip fractures in 65 women and 19 men in fluoridated communities and in 130 women and 32 men in nonfluoridated communities. The criteria for choosing the two nonfluoridated control areas were not presented, nor were hip fracture rates given separately for the two areas. That there might have been important differences between the exposed and nonexposed populations other than fluoridated drinking water is suggested by relative differences in their 1980 and 1987 populations. In the fluoridated community, the over-65 population decreased by 8% from 1980 to 1987, and in the two nonfluoridated areas, the over-65 population increased by 64% and 30%, respectively.

A geographic correlational study by Cooper et al. (1990, 1991) considered hip fracture hospital discharge rates in 39 urban areas of England,

9 of which had fluoridated water supplies and 30 of which did not. Initial analyses, which did not include adjustment for the precision of fracture rate estimates, did not find an association with fluoride concentrations in drinking water (R = 0.016, $p < 0.34$) (Cooper et al., 1990). However, in subsequent analyses, which used a weighted least-squares regression technique (weighting each district's rate estimate by the size of the population 45 years of age and older), a significant association between hip fracture discharge rate and fluoride concentration was found (R = 0.41, $p < 0.001$). As with Jacobsen et al. (1990), the use of this type of weighting in regression models might have placed too much emphasis on areas with large populations.

Skeletal Fluorosis

Finally, the subject of human skeletal fluorosis will be discussed briefly. Smith and Hodge (1979) have described the preclinical and clinical stages of skeletal fluorosis. The asymptomatic preclinical stage is characterized by slight increases in bone mass that are detectable radiographically and bone-ash fluoride concentrations between 3,500 and 5,500 ppm. The typical fluoride concentrations in bone ash from persons who have chronically consumed optimally fluoridated water are less than 1,500 ppm. In stage 1 of skeletal fluorosis, there might be occasional stiffness or pain in the joints and some osteosclerosis of the pelvis and vertebral column. Bone-ash fluoride concentrations in stage 1 usually range from 6,000 to 7,000 ppm. When bone-ash fluoride concentrations are 7,500-8,000 ppm or more, stages 2 and 3 of skeletal fluorosis are likely to occur. The clinical signs of these stages are chronic joint pain, dose-related calcification of ligaments, osteosclerosis, possibly osteoporosis of long bones, and in severe cases, muscle wasting and neurological defects.

Crippling skeletal fluorosis might occur in people who have ingested 10-20 mg of fluoride per day for 10-20 years. During the last 30 years, only five cases have been reported in the United States. The history of fluoride intake for two of the cases was determined with reasonable accuracy (Sauerbrunn et al., 1965; Goldman et al., 1971). The individuals consumed up to 6 L of water per day containing fluoride at 2.4-3.5 mg/L in one case and 4.0-7.8 mg/L in the other. The daily fluoride intake was estimated at 15-20 mg for 20 years. In general, this intake would be associated with a drinking-water supply containing fluoride at about 10 mg/L.

Thus, crippling skeletal fluorosis in the United States has been rare and not a public-health problem (Leone et al., 1954; Stevenson and Watson, 1957), even though for many generations there have been communities with drinking-water fluoride concentrations in excess of those that have resulted in the condition in other countries (Singh and Jolly, 1970). The puzzling geographic distribution of the disorder usually is ascribed to unidentified dietary factors that render the skeleton more or less susceptible.

The small number of cases of skeletal fluorosis in the United States has ruled out the possibility of systematic epidemiological evaluation. Based on limited data in the literature on skeletal fluorosis, the subcommittee concludes that skeletal fluorosis is not a public health issue in the United States.

Discussion

Of the six epidemiological studies that used geographic comparisons (where no actual intake data were available), four found a weak association between fluoride in drinking water and a small increase in the risk of hip (or other bone) fracture. In two of the four studies that observed associations, the weighting scheme for regression models might have been inappropriate. The risk increase in the positive studies was small. Of two additional studies that examined time trends in fracture rates before and after water fluoridation, one showed no association (Goggin et al., 1965) and the other found a negative association (Jacobsen et al., 1993). The time-trends ecological method is considered the stronger approach because there is less opportunity for confounding than in geographic comparison studies. Given the multiple limitations of ecological analyses, the possibility for publication bias in favor of positive findings and the potential in all the studies for confounding from factors common to all, these studies offer only limited support for a hypothesis of a weak association between fluoridated water and hip fracture, which requires confirmation in studies of individuals. Of the two studies with information on individuals, the analytical approach in one was essentially ecological (risk of hip fracture increased with fluoride at 4 mg/L of drinking water), and the other showed no difference in fracture risk in women who drank fluoridated or nonfluoridated water. In view of the conflicting results and limitations of the current data base on fluoride in drinking water and risk of hip or other fractures, there is no basis at this time to recommend that EPA lower the current maximum contaminant level (MCL) of fluoride of 4 mg/L.

The subcommittee recommends that additional studies of hip and other fractures be conducted in geographic areas with high and low concentrations of fluoride in drinking water, and that studies should use information from individuals rather than population groups. In these studies, it is important that individual information be collected about fluoride intake from drinking water and from all other sources, reproductive history, past and current hormonal status, intake of dietary and supplemental calcium and other cations, bone density, and other factors that might influence risk of fracture.

BONE FRACTURE IN ANIMALS

Studies with laboratory animals designed to determine the effects of fluoride on bone strength or fracture resistance have been done with several species, a variety of doses and periods of exposure, different stimuli to influence bone growth or resorption, and different measurement techniques. The associated bone fluoride concentrations have been documented in only some of the reports. The results of these studies on bone strength have yielded all possible outcomes (i.e., no effect, increased strength, decreased strength, and biphasic response). The most frequent finding, however, has been the absence of an effect. A representative sample of these reports will be discussed. The main features and findings of the studies are shown in Table 3-1.

Outcomes of studies showing a decrease in bone strength associated with high fluoride intake include those by Gedalia et al. (1964), Faccini (1969), and Wolinsky et al. (1972). Beary (1969) and Riggins et al. (1974) reported fluoride-associated decreases in bone strength in animals fed a calcium-deficient diet but not in animals fed a diet adequate in calcium.

In the study by Gedalia et al. (1964), weanling female "Sabra"-strain

TABLE 3-1 Effect of Fluoride on Bone Strength in Animals

Species, Sex, and Age	Water Fluoride,[a] mg/L, and Duration	Other	Bone-Ash Fluoride[b] ppm (Fluoride Group)	Stress Test	Findings	Reference
Rat, F, 20 d	0, 50; 4 wk	Estradiol, subcutaneous	Femur: 300 (0), 640 (50)	Bending	Strength reduced 25% in fluoride and fluoride + estradiol groups	Gedalia et al., 1964
Rabbit	200	None	Not reported	Not reported	Decreased strength	Faccini, 1969
Rat, M, 19 d	0, 200; 2 wk	None	Femur: 133 (0), 7,398 (200)	Bending	Strength reduced 38% in 200-mg/L group	Wolinsky et al., 1972
Rat, F, 25 d	0, 3, 10, 45; 3.5 mo	Adequate or low Ca diet	Femur: 5,000 (45; adequate Ca), 12,600 (45; low Ca)	Bending	No effect in adequate-Ca group; strength reduced in low-Ca, 10- and 45-mg/L fluoride groups	Beary, 1969
Rat, M, 4 wk	0, 50, 100; 3 mo	Adequate or low Ca diet	Tibia: 1,577 (50; adequate Ca), 7,393 (100; low Ca)	Torsion (femur)	No effect in adequate-Ca group; 28% reduction in strength only in low-Ca, 100-mg/L group	Riggins et al., 1974
Rat, M and F, 21 d	0, 1, 2, 4, 8, 16, 32, 64, 128; 16 wk	None	Vertebra: <1,000 (0-8), 1,500-11,000 (16-128)	Bending (femur)	Increased strength in 16-mg/L group; decreased strength in 64- and 128-mg/L groups (compared with 16-mg/L group)	Turner et al., 1992

Species	Dose (mg/L); duration	Diet/treatment	Bone fluoride (ppm)	Test	Results	Reference
Rat, F, 21 d	0, 5, 15, 30, 70; 16 wk	None	Vertebra: 75 (0), 750 (5), 2,500 (15), 5,400 (30), 10,600 (70)	Bending (femur)	Increased strength (26%) in 30-mg/L group; positive relation between strength and bone fluoride up to 5,400 ppm	Rich and Feist, 1970
Rat, M, 4 mo	0, 50; 30, 60 d	Suppl. Ca and vit. D for disuse osteoporosis	Tail vertebra: 1,324 at 30 d, 2,090 at 60 d	Compression	No effect on strength in groups with no disuse osteoporosis; increase in strength in osteoporosis + fluoride group	Rosen et al., 1975
Rat, M, 21 d	0, 50; 15 wk 0; 4, 8, 12 wk	Half received low Ca and low P diet after 15 wk	Femur: 4,000-5,000 at 15 wk	Bending	No effect in adequate-Ca and adequate-P group; fluoride did not prevent decrease in strength in low-Ca, low-P group	Kuo and Wuthier, 1975
Rat, M, 25 d	0, 2, 5, 20; up to 98 d	None	Not reported	Compression (femur and humerus)	No effect	Saville, 1967
Rat, 21 d	0, 10, 25, 100, 250; 13-52 wk	None	Not reported	Bending	No effect	Naylor and Wilson, 1967
Dog, Adult Beagle	0, 1, 3, 9, 27; 41 wk	Low Ca and high P diet to induce osteopenia	Femur cortical strips: 550 (0) to 1,800 (27)	Tension and bending	No effect	Romanus, 1974

TABLE 3-1 (Continued)

Species, Sex, and Age	Water Fluoride,[a] mg/L, and Duration	Other	Bone-Ash Fluoride[b] ppm (Fluoride Group)	Stress Test	Findings	Reference
Guinea pig, M, adult	0, 2, 10, 20; 15, 27, 42 wk	None	Rib, radius, and ulna: 660 (0 at 15 wk) to 3,560 (20 at 42 wk)	Tension, bending, and torsion (tibia, humerus, and femur)	No effect	Sharma et al., 1977
Rat, F, 21 d	25 (diet), 0, 11, 23, 34 (water); 86 d	None	Femur: 2,017 (0) to 11,688 (34)	Torsion (femur)	No effect	Einhorn et al., 1992
Bovine, F, 5-6 mo	0, 30, 50 (diet); 6 yr	None	Metacarpal: 595 (0), 2,664 (30), 4,500 (50)	Compression	No effect	Rahn et al., 1991

[a]Dietary fluoride (mg/kg) is noted in two studies.
[b]When bone fluoride was reported for dried bone, the fluoride was converted to milligrams per kilogram (parts per million) of bone ash, assuming an ash content of 60%.

rats were used. The rats were assigned to four groups: (1) untreated, (2) injected with estradiol twice weekly and given fluoridated water (50 mg/L), (3) injected with estradiol twice weekly and given nonfluoridated water, and (4) given fluoridated water without estradiol injections. The animals were killed after 4 weeks. The fluoride concentrations of femur ash in the untreated and estradiol groups were similar at about 300 ppm, and those of the fluoride-treated groups were 640 ppm. Compared with the untreated group, the average breaking strength (the force required to cause fracture), measured by bending, of the femurs was 22% higher in the estradiol-only group and about 25% lower in the fluoride-only and estradiol-fluoride groups.

In his review article of the effects of fluoride in bone, Faccini (1969) commented that a significant reduction in breaking strength of femurs occurred in rabbits that had received fluoride at 200 mg/L of drinking water for 8 weeks. No other details were provided.

Wolinsky et al. (1972) provided weanling male rats with food (fluoride at 5 mg/kg per day) and water containing no fluoride or fluoride at 200 mg/L per day for 2 weeks. The femur-ash fluoride concentrations were 133 ppm and 7,398 ppm, respectively. Femur strength was measured by bending and was found to be 38% lower in the fluoride-supplemented group.

Beary (1969) studied 25-day-old Sprague-Dawley rats that were given diets containing adequate (0.6%) or deficient (0.1%) amounts of calcium and drinking water that contained fluoride at 0, 3.4, 10, or 45 mg/L. After 15-16 weeks, femur strength was measured with the 3-point bending test. In the groups receiving adequate calcium, bone strength was slightly but not significantly lower in the fluoride-treated groups than in the untreated group, and a dose-response relation was not seen. Femur-shaft fluoride concentrations (calculated for ash content) ranged from 170 ppm in the control group to 5,000 ppm in the 45-mg/L group. In the calcium-deficient groups, fluoride-treated bone strength was reduced in a dose-dependent manner. Their bone fluoride concentrations were about twice as high as those in the groups receiving adequate calcium.

Riggins et al. (1974) used an experimental design similar to that of Beary's (1969), except that (1) the diet adequate in calcium contained 1.1% calcium, (2) drinking-water fluoride concentrations were 0, 50, and 100 mg/L, (3) fluoride exposure was 3 months, and (4) femur strength was measured by using fresh bones rapidly loaded in torsion, which was said to be "more analogous to the situation in which most long-bone fractures occur." Among the groups fed the 0.1%-calcium diet, bone strength was not affected in those receiving fluoride at 50 mg/L, but it was reduced by 28% in those at 100 mg/L. Tibia-ash fluoride concentrations in the 50- and 100-mg/L groups were 2,982 ppm and 7,393 ppm, respectively. In the groups fed the 1.1%-calcium diet, bone strength was not affected significantly by administration of fluoride. Tibia-ash fluoride concentrations in the control, 50-mg/L, and 100-mg/L groups were about 100, 1,580, and 5,200 ppm, respectively. Thus, as noted by Beary (1969), bone fluoride concentrations were significantly higher and breaking strengths were significantly lower in the calcium-deficient groups.

Turner et al. (1992) measured femur strength with the 3-point bending test and reported a biphasic response to the concentration of fluoride intake. Nine groups of weanling rats received a low-fluoride diet (less than 2 mg/kg per day) and water containing fluoride at 0-128 mg/L for 16 weeks. For reasons that are not clear, the range of bone fluoride concentrations (vertebral ash) in all nine groups was unusually high. As a result, average values were difficult to determine accurately. Nevertheless, average values were less than 1,000 ppm for the groups receiving fluoride at 0-8 mg/L (bone fluoride at about 100 ppm), and there was no difference in bone strength among them. The 16-mg/L group had an average bone fluoride concentration of about 1,500 ppm and an increase in strength that was significantly higher than that in the 0-, 1-, 8-, 64-, and 128-mg/L groups. The average femur fluoride concentrations of the 64- and 128-mg/L groups were about 5,000 and 11,000 ppm, respectively. The bone strengths of these groups were lower than those of all other groups, but the differences were statistically significant only when compared with the 16-mg/L group. Because the difference between bone strength in the 64- and 128-mg/L groups and the 1- and 8-mg/L groups was not statistically significant, however, the authors' interpretation of a "biphasic response" appears tenuous.

Rich and Feist (1970) provided pregnant rats with a low-fluoride diet during the last 5 days before delivery and during the nursing period in an effort to reduce the bone fluoride concentrations of the offspring. Sixty female weanling pups were then assigned to five groups that received drinking water containing fluoride at 0, 5, 15, 30, or 70 mg/L for 16 weeks. The breaking strengths of femurs were determined with a 3-point bending test, and the fluoride concentrations of the second lumbar vertebrae were determined with the ion-specific electrode. The breaking strength of the femurs in the 30-mg/L group was 26% higher ($p < 0.01$) than the breaking strength of the control group. None of the other groups differed from the control group in breaking strength, but as determined by linear regression analysis, there was a positive relation ($p < 0.01$) between bone fluoride concentration and breaking strength in the 0-, 5-, 15- and 30-mg/L groups. The strength of the regression was not affected significantly by differences in body weight, bone weight, bone length, bone diameter, or cortical thickness. The bone fluoride concentrations ranged from 75 to 5,400 ppm in those groups. Although the bone fluoride concentration (calculated in terms of ash) of the 70-mg/L group was 10,580 ppm, the breaking strength was not significantly different from that of the 0-mg/L group (14.2 vs. 13.1 kg, respectively).

Rosen et al. (1975) noted an increase in vertebral bone strength associated with increased fluoride intake in rats with disuse osteoporosis. Their study involved adult male Sabra-strain rats. The tails of one-half of the rats were surgically immobilized to induce disuse osteoporosis. The four subgroups received distilled drinking water, fluoride at 50 mg/L of drinking water, distilled drinking water and supplemental calcium and vitamin D, and fluoride at 50 mg/L of drinking water for 30 days followed by distilled drinking water and supplemental calcium and vitamin D for 30 days. The study lasted 60 days. The compressive strength of the tail vertebrae did not differ among the groups whose tails were not immobilized. In the groups with disuse osteoporosis, bone strength was increased by about 30% with fluoride administration and also by 15% with supplemental calcium and vitamin D administration. The average bone-ash fluoride concentration of the groups that did not receive supplemental fluoride was 440 ppm, and the concentrations of the 50-mg/L groups were 2,090 ppm (60 days on fluoridated water) and 1,324 ppm (30 days on fluoridated water).

Studies showing no effect of fluoride administration on bone strength have involved rats (Saville, 1967; Naylor and Wilson, 1967; Kuo and Wuthier, 1975; Einhorn et al., 1992), dogs (Romanus, 1974), guinea pigs (Sharma et al., 1977), and cows (Rahn et al., 1991). Kuo and Wuthier (1975) used weanling male Sprague-Dawley rats in their study to determine the possible preventive effects of fluoride in diet-induced osteoporosis. The rats were fed a nutritionally adequate diet with or without fluoride at 50 mg/L of drinking water for 15 weeks, at which time 6-7 rats were killed to provide baseline data. One-half of the remaining rats in each group continued to receive the nutritionally adequate diet and the others were given a low-calcium (0.014%) and phosphorus (0.018%) diet. All rats were then given distilled water without fluoride to drink until they were killed 4, 8, or 12 weeks later. The baseline (15-week) fluoride concentrations of femur ash were 4,000-5,000 ppm in the 50-mg/L group and 50-60 ppm in the control group. There was no difference between the 0- and 50-mg/L groups in bone strength at that time. The concentrations were said to "gradually increase" thereafter but at a "significantly greater rate" in rats receiving the low-calcium, phosphorus diet. This diet caused a progressive loss of bone mass and an important decrease in mid-shaft femur strength. Fluoride administration, however, had no effect on these changes.

Saville (1967) assigned 25-day-old Charles River CD-strain male rats to four groups that received fluoride at 0, 2, 5, or 20 mg/L of drinking water. The rats were killed at selected times up to 98 days. The compressive strength of the femurs and humeri was determined and found to be a linear function of body weight but did not differ among the groups. Naylor and Wilson (1967) performed a similar study with weanling albino rats but with higher drinking-water fluoride concentrations (0, 10, 25, 100, or 250 mg/L) for up to 52 weeks. No differences were found among the groups in radiographic appearance, breaking strength, deflexion pattern on bending, or ash content of femurs. These two reports did not contain bone fluoride concentrations.

Romanus (1974) examined physical properties and chemical composition of canine (Beagles) femoral cortical bone strips after nutritional osteopenia was induced by feeding a low-calcium, high-phosphorus diet for 41 weeks. Fluoride was added to the diet at 0, 1, 3, 9, or 27 mg/kg. The same analyses done on bone samples obtained from dogs were continued in the study to test for "reversibility." This involved feeding a diet enriched in calcium and phosphorus for up to 28 additional weeks. The physical properties of bone were determined with 3- and 4-point bending tests and application of tension. Dietary fluoride supplementation had no effect on the composition of bone (except for a direct correlation with bone fluoride concentrations). Similarly, bone strength was not affected significantly by administration of fluoride. The author offered a concluding comment: "A better source for studies of bone is bone from individuals with skeletal disease, as nutritional and disuse osteopenia does not seem to change the physical properties of the bone material to any major extent."

Sharma et al. (1977) assigned adult male Hartley guinea pigs to four groups that were given distilled drinking water containing fluoride at 0, 2, 10, or 20 mg/L. The Purina diet was stated to contain fluoride at less than 17 mg/kg. This diet was a "maintenance" diet, so that the bioavailability of fluoride would have been approximately 50% (Whitford, 1991). Thus, there was no true low-fluoride group. The animals were killed at 15, 27, or 42 weeks. The physical properties of selected long bones were determined with tension, bending, and torsion tests. The fluoride concentrations of rib, radius, and ulna were directly related to time of fluoride exposure and to concentration of fluoride exposure. After 42 weeks, the fluoride concentrations of the bones (dry) in the 20-mg/L group were 2,565, 1,990 and 1,855 ppm, which would correspond to an average concentration of 3,560 ppm in bone ash. There were no statistically significant differences among the groups with respect to tension strength (fracture upon pulling), torsion modulus (fracture upon twisting), or modulus of elasticity (fracture upon bending).

Einhorn et al. (1992) provided weanling female rats with a maintenance diet containing fluoride at 25 mg/kg and drinking water with fluoride at 0, 11, 23, or 34 mg/L for 86 days. As in several of the other studies, this study did not have a low-fluoride group. The average femur-ash fluoride concentrations for these groups were 2,017, 6,102, 9,097 and 11,688 ppm, respectively. The torsional strength of the femurs did not differ among the groups. In agreement with Riggins et al. (1974), it was stated that testing animal bones in torsion is more akin to the stress pattern most often encountered by human patients. Einhorn et al. also examined bone with histomorphometric techniques and found no significant intergroup differences. They concluded that, in the absence of effects on bone mass, remodeling, or formation rate, incorporation of even very high concentrations of fluoride does not significantly alter the capacity of bone to withstand mechanical loads.

Rahn et al. (1991) assigned 17 Holstein heifer calves 5-6 months old to three groups fed a diet containing fluoride at 0, 30, or 50 mg/kg. The fluoride concentration of the control diet was not stated but must have been fairly low because of the bone fluoride concentrations. The experimental groups received fluoride at 0.5-1.2 mg/kg per day or 0.8-1.8 mg/kg per day. After 6 years, the metacarpal bones were analyzed for fluoride, density, and compressive strength. The bone-ash fluoride concentrations were 595, 2,664, and 4,500 ppm in the 0-, 30-, and 50-mg/L groups, respectively. The relation between bone density and fluoride concentration appeared to be inverse, but the trend was not statistically significant. Compressive strength did not differ among the groups.

Discussion

The results of the laboratory animal studies designed to determine the effects of fluoride administration on bone strength have yielded all possible outcomes. Although most of the reports indicate little or no effect even with extremely high fluoride intake and bone concentrations, some have shown positive, negative, or biphasic effects. The explanations for these discrepant results are not apparent. Several potential or real problems in experimental design, however, have been identified. Insofar as can be determined, only three of the studies used a diet with a reasonably low fluoride concentration (Rich and Feist, 1970; Rahn et al., 1991; Turner et al., 1992) and most used diets with frankly high concentrations. Consequently, the control groups in the latter studies often had high concentrations of bone fluoride, which could have obscured positive or negative effects on bone strength in the treatment groups. That is to say, when diets with high fluoride concentrations are used and bone fluoride concentrations in the control groups are clearly high, no true low-fluoride group exists that can be used to judge the effects of fluoride in the treatment groups. In the three studies that used low-fluoride diets, the investigators found that bone strength was not affected or was actually increased in one or more of the treatment groups.

Another problem in some of the reports is the method used for determining bone fluoride. For example, Beary (1969) said that the solution of bone mineral to be analyzed was adjusted to a pH of "2.07 $\pm$ 0.03 since this is considered a desirable range for reading fluoride ion activity" with the fluoride electrode. The pH range actually recommended is 5-6. This range is well above the pK of hydrogen fluoride (3.4), which is not "seen" by the electrode but is sufficiently low so that hydroxyl ions do not interfere (the electrode recognizes both fluoride and hydroxyl ions). At a pH of 2.07, only 5% of the fluoride in solution is detectable by the electrode. Other investigators dissolved the bone samples in strong acid while the vessels were open to the air. The boiling point of hydrofluoric acid is 19°C, so fluoride loss from the sample might have occurred. The hexamethyldisiloxane-facilitated diffusion method of Taves (1968), as modified by Whitford (1989), is a preparative technique that has been shown to be reliable and accurate.

The subcommittee concludes that the weight of evidence currently available indicates that bone strength in animals fed a nutritionally adequate diet is not adversely affected unless chronic exposure to fluoride is at least 50 mg/kg in diet or 50 mg/L in water. These data indicate that the current EPA guidelines of fluoride at 4 mg/L of drinking water for humans are appropriate. Recent reports from epidemiological studies of human populations have provided conflicting evidence on this subject, however, and indicate the need for additional research.

One uncertainty in all the studies is the appropriateness of the methods used to cause bone fractures. Most investigators have used a bending test, although torsion, tension, or compression tests have also been used. Compression tests would be appropriate for vertebrae but rarely for long bones. Pure tension stress would almost never be involved in the fracture of any human bone. Bending has a torsional component, but forces are applied to specific points that might not reflect the overall strength of the bone. Torsion gives a uniform strain field that might yield a more realistic estimate of the load required to cause fracture. According to Riggins et al. (1974) and Einhorn et al. (1992), torsion or twisting is most analogous to the stress experienced by humans who have fractures of long bones.

To resolve the uncertainties that surround this important area of investigation, the subcommittee recommends that a workshop be conducted to evaluate the advantages and disadvantages of the various doses, treatments, laboratory animal models, weight-bearing versus non-weight-bearing bones, and testing methods for bone strength that can be used to determine the effects of fluoride on bone.

4

REPRODUCTIVE EFFECTS OF FLUORIDE

REPRODUCTIVE EFFECTS IN HUMANS

There are no published reports in the literature on reproductive toxicity of fluoride in men. However, two Russian studies showed that chronic occupational exposure to fluoride-contaminated compounds might affect reproductive function. Men who had worked in the cryolite industry for 10-25 years and who demonstrated clinical skeletal fluorosis showed decreases in circulating testosterone and compensatory increases in follicle-stimulating hormone when compared with controls (Tokar and Savchenko, 1977). Of the exposed men, those exposed to cryolite for 16-25 years had increased luteinizing-hormone levels as compared with men exposed for 10-15 years. Women exposed occupationally to air heavily laden with superphosphates demonstrated increases in menstrual irregularities and genital irritations when compared with unexposed controls (Kuznetzova, 1969). However, occupational exposure to many other compounds in the cryolite and superphosphate industries makes it difficult to implicate any one substance, such as fluoride, in inducing these health effects.

A recent study of women employed in silicon wafer manufacturing (fabrication room workers) showed a relative risk of spontaneous abortions of 1.45 times that of women (of the same ages) who worked in nonfabrication rooms (Schenker et al., 1992). The overall increase in

73

risk ranged from about 20% to 40%. There was a dose-response relationship and a consistency of findings for persons exposed to one specific class of solvents. Spontaneous abortions were also associated with fluoride exposure but only in one work group, and a strong dose-response was not present. The authors characterized the fluoride-associated increase in relative risk of spontaneous abortions as "less consistent" than the results of exposure to some solvents in this study and "less consistent" with other research.

REPRODUCTIVE EFFECTS IN ANIMALS

A summary of the reproductive effects of fluoride in animals is presented in Table 4-1. Several of the earliest studies of the effects in rodents noted an adverse effect when the diet contained fluoride at more than 100 mg/kg. Phillips et al. (1933) concluded that the upper limit of safety of chronic intake of fluoride by the rat in terms of effects on estrus cycle, rate of reproduction, and lactation was 20 mg/kg of body weight per day. In their study, fluoride was added to the diet as sodium fluoride (190 mg/kg) or rock phosphate (sodium fluoride at 210 and 350 mg/kg). The fluoride concentration of the stock diet, which also contained bone meal, was not stated. Most "natural ingredient" rodent diets containing bone meal that are available today, however, have fluoride concentrations ranging from 10 to 50 mg/kg. The bioavailability of fluoride from these diets is 45-50% (Whitford, 1991).

In their study of the effects of fluoride on the reproductive performance of male rats, Araibi et al. (1989) added fluoride at 0, 100, or 200 mg/kg to the "standard" rat diet. The fluoride concentration of the standard diet was not reported. After 60 days, blood was collected from some of the rats for determination of testosterone concentration, and the testes were prepared for microscopic examination. The fertility of the remaining rats was tested by mating them with normal females for 4 days. The number of pregnancies and offspring was reduced significantly in the 200-mg/kg group but not in the 100-mg/kg group. The litter sizes did not differ among any of the groups. The authors commented that the treated rats showed "less interest toward females." However, food and water intakes, body-weight changes, and activity levels were not reported and were probably reduced in the 200-mg/kg group. If so, those effects might have been involved in the apparent loss of interest. The diameters of the seminiferous tubules were reduced slightly in both fluoride-treated groups. The thickness of the peritubular membranes was increased, the percentage of tubules with spermatozoa was reduced, and the serum testosterone level was lower in the 200-mg/kg group. Those effects did not occur in the 100-mg/kg group.

Messer et al. (1973) fed mice a low-fluoride diet (0.1-0.3 mg/kg) and drinking water containing fluoride at 0, 50, 100, or 200 mg/L for 33 weeks. The two highest amounts resulted in retarded growth and impaired reproduction; increased mortality occurred in the 200-mg/L group only. No litters were produced by mice in the 200-mg/L group, and only nine litters were born to the 50 mice in the 100-mg/L group. Six of the nine litters were stillborn or eaten at birth. Litter production in the 50-mg/L group was normal. The fluoride concentrations in ashed humeri were about 100 ppm in the control group and 7,800 ppm in the 50-mg/L group. According to Messer et al., the group that received no fluoride showed signs of "fluorine deficiency with a progressive development of infertility in two successive generations." That finding was based on the development of anemia and the fact that fewer litters were produced in the control group than in the 50-mg/L group. The authors concluded that their findings supported the necessity of fluoride in the diet of mice.

Tao and Suttie (1976) repeated the study of Messer et al. (1973) as closely as possible, except that the diet contained adequate levels of iron and copper and fluoride was added to the diet at concentrations of 2 and 100 mg/kg. The stock diet had a fluoride concentration of less than 0.5 mg/kg. Femur-ash fluoride concentrations of the third-generation mice in the 0-, 2-, and 100-mg/kg groups at 33 weeks were 90, 328, and 10,020 ppm, respectively. The investigators noted no differences among the groups with respect to hematocrit or reproduction. They concluded that the fluoride-deficiency findings of Messer et al. (1973) were probably due to an iron or copper deficiency. The role of fluoride was considered secondary in that it prevented fluoride deficiency from developing, apparently by increasing the absorption of iron and copper, both of which were present in marginal concentrations in Messer's mouse diet.

Studies of reproduction in cattle have generally shown no effect of fluoride unless intake is sufficient to produce skeletal fluorosis and other adverse effects. The reports by Phillips et al. (1934) and Mitchell and Edman (1952) indicated that reproductive performance of cattle with

TABLE 4-1 Reproductive Effects of Fluoride in Experimental Animals

Species	Water or Diet Fluoride or Fluoride Dose	Duration	Bone-Ash Fluoride[a] (Fluoride Group)	Findings	Reference
Rat	0 or 190 mg/kg as NaF; 210 or 350 mg/kg as rock phosphate	5 generations	Not reported	No effects until dose exceeded 20 mg/kg/day	Phillips et al., 1933
Rat	0, 100, 200 mg/kg	60 d	Not reported	Reduced fertility, spermatogenesis, and serum testosterone in 200-mg/kg group	Araibi et al., 1989
Mouse	0, 50, 100, 200 mg/L	33 wk	100 (0), 7,800 (50)	Impaired litter production in 100- and 200-mg/L groups; diet was marginal in Fe and Cu	Messer et al., 1973
Mouse	0, 2, 100 mg/kg	33 wk	90 (0), 328 (2), 10,020 (100)	No effect; diet was adequate in Fe and Cu	Tao and Suttie, 1976
Bovine	0, 0.75, 1.5 mg/kg	74-77 mo	552-15,200 (0 and 1.5)	No effect, except marginal reduction in milk production	Suttie et al., 1972
Bovine	5, 8, 12 mg/L with or without superphosphate added to diet	4 breeding seasons	Not reported	Delayed estrus, reduced fertility in 8- and 12-mg/L groups, especially superphosphate groups	van Rensburg and de Vos, 1966
Bovine	97 mg/kg in commercial concentrate; 1,415 mg/kg in mineral mix	6 yr	300 in 2-yr-old to 2,100 in 6-yr-old	Problems with general health, reproduction, and milk production	Eckerlin et al., 1986a
Owl	0, 40, 200 mg/kg	5-6 mo	Not reported	No effect on egg production, slight decrease in egg volume in 40- and 200-mg/kg groups	Hoffman et al., 1985

Owl	0, 40, 200 mg/kg	5-6 mo	Not reported	No effect on nesting chronology, clutch size, percent fertility, or percent of eggs hatched of those incubated; number of young per clutch lower in 200-mg/kg group	Pattee et al., 1988
Hen	0-1,300 mg/kg	112 d	Not reported	Improved egg production in 200-mg/kg group, no effect on fertility or hatchability, egg size reduced at >1,000 ppm	Guenter, 1979
Kestrel	62, 4,513, 7,691 mg/kg	10 d	261 (62), 730 (4,513), 798 (7,691)	No effect on clutch size, fertility, or hatchability	Carriere et al., 1987
Mink	0, 33, 60, 108, 194, 350 mg/kg	382 d	1,362 (0), 3,511 (33), 5,202 (60), 6,425 (108) 9,177 (194), 13,706 (350)	No effect on breeding, gestation, whelping, or lactation	Aulerich et al., 1987
Fox	98-137 mg/kg		500-900 in kits, 2,000-3,000 in adults	Reduced milk production, starvation of kits	Eckerlin et al., 1986b
Fox	8-23 mg/kg	2 yr	222 in 9-mo-old foxes, 1,379 in adults	Problems reported in 1986 were ameliorated after changing to low-fluoride diet	Eckerlin et al., 1988
Dog	0-460 mg/kg	2 yr	Not reported	No convincing evidence of fluoride-induced reproductive effects	Schellenberg et al, 1990

[a]Bone fluoride concentrations expressed as milligrams per kilogram (parts per million) of bone ash.

signs of chronic fluorosis was unaffected except for delays in estrus after parturition. Suttie et al. (1972) exposed Holstein heifers to different patterns of dietary fluoride for 6 years. The fluoride doses ranged from that contained only in the forage and grain to supplements of 3.0 mg/kg per day for 4 months, alternating with 0.75 mg/kg per day for 8 months. On an annual basis, the doses given to the fluoride-treated groups were 0.75 and 1.5 mg/kg per day. At the end of the study, the fluoride concentration in vertebral ash was 552 ppm in the control group, and the concentrations ranged from 7,660 to 15,200 ppm in the treatment groups. Skeletal fluorosis was evident in all treatment groups. The authors concluded that no differences existed among the groups in growth rate or reproductive performance, although "the conception rate for the entire experiment was low." Milk production was "somewhat less" in animals receiving 1.5 mg/kg per day each year, "but as small numbers of animals were involved, the observations are inconclusive."

In their study, van Rensburg and de Vos (1966) noted the effects of fluoride on reproductive performance of Afrikaner heifers receiving fluoride at 5-12 mg/L of drinking water. Five groups were given drinking water containing fluoride at 5 or 8 mg/L or fluoride at 5, 8, or 12 mg/L and superphosphate (chiefly tribasic calcium phosphate produced by treating phosphate rock with sulfuric acid), which had been treated to reduce its fluoride content. The fluoride concentrations in food, superphosphate, or drinking water after addition of superphosphate were not stated. No group was given nonfluoridated water, and fluoride concentrations in bone or other tissues were not determined. Breeding was started 9 months after beginning exposure to fluoride and observations on reproductive performance were made over four breeding seasons. The heifers were bred naturally during the first two breeding seasons and by artificial insemination during the last two seasons. Reproduction did not differ among the groups during the first season. In the second season, anestrus after parturition increased in the 8- and 12-mg/L groups. In the third season, fertility clearly declined in those two groups but was more pronounced in the superphosphate groups. In the fourth season, the effects were even greater as judged by the calving rates and the services per conception in all groups, especially in the 8- and 12-mg/L groups that were given superphosphate. Contrary to what was expected, the addition of superphosphate to the water aggravated the effects of fluoride, which suggested to the authors that the removal of fluoride might have been incomplete and that actual fluoride intakes were more than had been intended. Despite those uncertainties, it was concluded that "for normal reproduction the fluorine content of the drinking water should be under 5 mg/L."

Eckerlin et al. (1986a) reported on a problem with milk production on a dairy farm. From January 1977 through August 1978, the average annual milk yield was 7,851 kg per cow per year. The fluoride concentration of the diet used during that period was not reported. In September 1978, a new commercial concentrate and mineral mix was introduced as a supplement to the diet. During the next 6 years, problems developed in the general health, reproduction, and milk production of the cows. The average fluoride concentration of three bags of the concentrate saved from 1982 was 97 mg/kg. One sample of the mineral mix from 1982 had a fluoride content of 1,415 mg/kg. Milk production during 1978-1984 averaged 5,434 kg per cow per year, a decline of 31%. When the investigators conducted their study at the farm in 1984, the last ossified coccygeal vertebrae of 15 cows were surgically removed and analyzed for fluoride. The fluoride concentrations in bone ash ranged from 300 ppm in a 2-year-old cow to 2,100 ppm in a 6-year-old cow. Considering the adverse effects that were recorded and the reportedly high concentrations of fluoride in the diet, those values were very low. The low fluoride concentrations in bone do not support the contention that the effects were due to fluoride toxicity. As noted above, Suttie et al. (1972) found bone fluoride concentrations of over 15,000 ppm and essentially none of the toxic manifestations reported by Eckerlin et al. (1986a).

Other studies of the effects of fluoride on reproduction in owls, hens, kestrels, dogs, and mink have been reported. Hoffman et al. (1985) and Pattee et al. (1988) provided a diet supplemented with fluoride at 0, 40, or 200 mg/kg to breeding pairs of screech owls (60 and 33 pairs, respectively) for 5-6 months. The control diet had a fluoride concentration of 27.2 mg/kg. In the Hoffman et al. study, no differences were found in the number of eggs laid by all the groups. Egg volume was 6% lower in two of the treatment groups. Five hatchlings weighed slightly less in the 40-mg/kg group and 9% weighed slightly less in the 200-mg/kg group than in the control group, but this difference disappeared 7 days later. Pattee et al. (1988) reported that nesting chronology was similar among all groups with respect to initiation of egg laying, initiation of incubation, hatching date, intervals between any of those events, clutch size, percent fertility, and percent of eggs hatched. The number of young produced per clutch was lower in the 200-mg/kg group than in the control group (2.6 ± 0.4 vs. 4.2 ± 0.4). Congenital anomalies were not observed in either study, nor were the concentrations of fluoride in bone. However, Pattee et al. (1988) reported the fluoride concentrations in eggshell ash. The eggshell concentrations of the control, 40-, and 200-mg/kg groups were 6.4 ppm, 53 ppm, and 87 ppm, respectively. It was of interest that the differences in the 40- and 200-mg/kg groups were not statistically significant. The authors concluded that slight-to-moderate reproduction disorders in screech owls (slightly lower egg volume and initial body weight) might occur in areas heavily polluted with fluoride.

Guenter (1979) fed chickens diets containing fluoride at 0-1,300 mg/kg. The results suggested that dietary fluoride at 200 mg/kg per day for 112 days improved egg production and feed efficiency, although shell thickness was reduced slightly. Dietary fluoride had no effect on fertility or hatchability of chicken eggs. In a second experiment, dietary fluoride at 100 mg/kg improved feed efficiency, shell quality, and the number of collectible eggs. Egg size was reduced only in the groups fed fluoride at 1,000 mg/kg and 1,300 mg/kg. Calcified-tissue fluoride concentrations were not reported.

The effects on reproduction in 24 pairs of American kestrels fed cockerels with a low or high fluoride content for 10 days were reported by Carriere et al. (1987). The cockerels fed to the control group had a background femur fluoride concentration of 62 ppm and those fed to the treatment groups had concentrations of 4,513 ppm and 7,691 ppm. Femur fluoride concentrations of the kestrels were proportional to fluoride intake. The clutch sizes tended to be smaller as the concentration of fluoride intake increased, but the differences were not statistically significant. Percent fertility and percent hatchability were not related to fluoride intake.

Pastel mink were fed diets supplemented with fluoride at 0, 33, 60, 108, 194, or 350 mg/kg per day for 382 days (Aulerich et al., 1987). The fluoride concentration of the nonsupplemented diet was 35 mg/kg. There were no important differences among the groups in breeding, gestation, whelping, or lactation. The survivability of kits whelped by minks fed fluoride at 350 mg/kg was markedly decreased. The body weights of those whelped by minks in the 60- and 108-mg/kg groups were higher than those of the control group at 3 and 6 weeks. The femur fluoride concentrations of the six groups were directly related to the fluoride dose and ranged from 1,362 to 13,706 ppm.

Eckerlin et al. (1986b) reported a problem with milk production and survival rates of kits at three fox farms. The farms had successfully produced pelts for several years. In 1985, the foxes experienced severe early postpartum agalactia, which resulted in high mortality of kits during the first few postpartum days. Analysis of the commercial diets used on the three farms revealed fluoride concentrations of 98-137 mg/kg. Control diets from another supplier had fluoride concentrations of 23 and 31 mg/kg. Bone fluoride concentrations increased with age from about 500-900 ppm in the kits to 2,000-3,000 ppm in the adults. The authors concluded that the agalactia was caused by excessive fluoride intake. Reduced milk production associated with high fluoride intake has also been reported for cows (Maylin and Krook, 1982), although, as reported above, Suttie et al. (1972) reported only a marginal effect in cows that were exposed to high fluoride doses.

In a followup study at the fox farm, Eckerlin et al. (1988) provided additional evidence that the problems were related to high fluoride concentrations in the diets. The fluoride concentrations of new diets used from 1985 to 1987 ranged from 8 to 23 mg/kg. Bone fluoride concentrations declined, kit production increased, and kit survivability approached normal expectations.

From 1970 to 1980, an increased incidence of perinatal deaths and congenital deformities occurred in a kennel of Shetland sheepdogs (Schellenberg et al., 1990). The problems started shortly after the kennel was moved from an old frame building to a new concrete-block building. In 1979 and 1980, mottled teeth in the few surviving pups and cranial exostoses in the adults were noted for the first time. These calcified-tissue effects were attributed to the high fluoride content of the diet (460 mg/kg added in the form of rock phosphate).

In 1982, a 2-year study of 20 shelties of proven fertility was started to determine the reproductive effects of high-fluoride diet and kennel well water (Schellenberg et al., 1990). The well water was of interest after it became clear that some unknown factor in the kennel environment was responsible for the adverse reproductive effects. There were four treatment groups (four females and one male in each group) that were given a high- or low-fluoride diet (55 mg/kg) and kennel well water or distilled water. Except for the group fed the low-fluoride diet and well water (which produced the expected number of pups), the number of pups whelped in the other groups paralleled the poor reproduction results that prompted the study. The two high-fluoride groups produced only two litters and 15 pups, 10 (67%) of which were dead within 7 days. The two low-fluoride groups produced six litters and 33 pups, 14 (42%) of which were dead within the first 7 postpartum days. The two well-water groups produced six litters and 39 pups, 18 (46%) of which died within 7 days. The two distilled-water groups produced two litters and 9 pups, 5 (56%) of which died within 7 days. It was determined that the perinatal deaths were not due to agalactia. Overall, the missed pregnancy rate was 44% and the perinatal death rate was 50%. No serious congenital defects occurred in the high-fluoride groups and two occurred in the low-fluoride groups. Several minor congenital defects occurred in all groups. The authors concluded that, "Although 460 mg/kg F in the dog food did produce bony exostoses, we did not find convincing evidence that it adversely affected reproduction in shelties. The cause of the reproductive problems was apparently not the dog food, water, foliage, genetic factors, or infectious disease and currently remains undetermined."

The problem was further examined in a study using rats (Marks et al., 1984). Four treatment groups (9 males and 18 females in each group) were given the same diet of dog food containing fluoride at 460 or 55 mg/kg and the same sources of drinking water as described above. The rats were brought into the kennel at 39 days of age, given the specified diets for the next 60 days, and then mated. The authors concluded that "even after two litters, the only adverse effect was dental fluorosis in the high-fluoride groups. The results indicated that rats cannot be used in the search for the cause(s) of reproductive problems in dogs in this kennel."

DISCUSSION

Adverse effects on reproductive performance associated with high concentrations of fluoride intake have been demonstrated in mice, rats, cattle, owls, hens, kestrels, dogs, mink, and foxes (reduced lactation). The water or food threshold fluoride concentration associated with these effects in mice, rats, cattle, and foxes is approximately 100 mg/L (100 mg/kg). An exception to this was reported by van Rensburg and de Vos

(1966) who concluded that the water fluoride concentration should be less than 5 mg/L for normal reproduction in cattle. The authors noted, however, that the fluoride concentration in the superphosphate added to three of the five diets was not known, so the actual concentrations of fluoride in those diets might have been higher than intended. The threshold concentration for mink, owls, and kestrels is 100-200 mg/kg and for hens over 500 mg/kg in diet. These dietary fluoride concentrations are much higher than those in the fluoridated drinking water of humans. This fact is consistent with the lack of evidence suggesting a link between consumption of fluoridated water and problems with human reproduction.

It was noted in several of the studies outlined above that the fluoride concentrations in the diets of the control groups were unknown or considerably higher than is optimal. In these cases, the investigators might not have been able to detect the effects, if any, of fluoride intake at the low end of the dosage scale. It is recommended that future studies of reproductive effects of fluoride intake include control diets with fluoride concentrations of less than 1.0 mg/kg. To confirm the level of fluoride exposure, it is also recommended that bone fluoride concentrations be measured using accurate and reliable preparative and analytical methods, such as the hexamethyldisiloxane-facilitated diffusion method of Taves (1968) as modified by Whitford (1989) and the fluoride ion-specific electrode.

5 EFFECTS OF INGESTED FLUORIDE ON RENAL, GASTROINTESTESTINAL, AND IMMUNE SYSTEMS

EFFECTS ON THE RENAL SYSTEM

The kidney is the potential site of acute fluoride toxicity because kidney cells are exposed to relatively high fluoride concentrations. Fluoride concentrations in the kidney show an increasing gradient of concentration, the lowest concentrations occurring in the renal cortex and the highest in the papilla (Whitford, 1990). Fluoride, after oral administration, is rapidly absorbed into the blood. Peak serum concentrations occur 30-90 minutes after administration and then decline rapidly (Cowell and Taylor, 1981). Approximately 50% of the daily intake of fluoride is cleared by the kidneys (Whitford, 1990). Consequently, the kidney is thought to be a target organ for any adverse effects of fluoride because of the bioconcentration and kinetics of fluoride metabolism and excretion patterns.

A few experimental studies have examined the effects of fluoride exposure on rodent kidneys. Daston et al. (1985) administered a single intraperitoneal dose of fluoride at 30 or 40 mg/kg of body weight to 29-day-old rats. They observed transitory (disappearing within 120 hours) renal effects, such as polyuria, increased urinary pH, and proximal tubular cell necrosis. The renal effects in rodents are probably age-dependent because suckling rats have a lower urinary pH than weanling rats do. The lower pH likely results in more selective reabsorption of

85

fluoride, which results in higher tissue concentrations. Studies of weanling rats consuming water with high concentrations of sodium fluoride (NaF at 380 mg/L for 6 weeks) have demonstrated necrosis of the proximal and distal renal tubules (Lim et al., 1978). In a study of weanling rats administered drinking water with NaF at 100 mg/L for 6 months, Taylor et al. (1961) reported interstitial nephritis and dilation of the renal tubules at the corticomedullary junction. No effects were observed at 50 mg/L. Structural changes in the kidneys have also been reported by other investigators following chronic fluoride exposure, although the eventual effects on renal function were not examined (Hodge and Smith, 1977; Greenberg, 1986).

In humans, the potential for health effects of fluoride exposures on renal function is enhanced because of selective absorption by the kidney and the kinetics of fluoride distribution and excretion. The healthy kidney removes fluoride from the blood much more efficiently than it removes the other halogens. Furthermore, the tissue-to-plasma fluoride-concentration ratios for soft tissues were highest in the kidneys (Whitford, 1989). Studies of persons receiving the halogenated anesthesia, methoxyflurane, observed renal insufficiency in some patients due to high serum fluoride concentrations (Mazze, 1984). The effect was transient, and renal function returned to normal once the serum fluoride concentrations decreased below 30 micromoles (μmol)/L. Several epidemiological studies have examined the possible association between fluoride exposures and renal effects. Hanhijarvi (1975), in a study of plasma fluoride concentrations in 2,200 hospital patients in Finland (which included 501 persons living in an area with naturally occurring fluoride concentrations at less than 0.2 mg/L of drinking water and 1,083 persons living in an area with fluoride added to drinking water at 1 mg/L), showed that concentrations increased with age and were higher in individuals living in the area with added fluoride in drinking water. Renal clearance of fluoride increased with age in both groups but was approximately twice as high in persons living in the area with added fluoride. Decreased renal clearance of fluoride was observed in persons with renal insufficiency or with diabetes mellitus. Other studies have shown decreased fluoride clearance in both adults and children with impaired renal function (Kono et al., 1984; Spak et al., 1985). Several large community-based epidemiological studies found no increased renal disease associated with long-term exposure to drinking water with fluoride concentrations up to 8 mg/L (Leone et al., 1954; Schlesinger et al., 1956; Geever et al., 1958).

In summary, although experimental studies have shown transient and permanent renal effects at concentrations of fluoride over 50-100 mg/L, human epidemiological studies have not observed increased renal disease in populations with long-term exposure to fluoride concentrations up to 8 mg/L of drinking water.

EFFECTS ON THE GASTROINTESTINAL SYSTEM

With the exception of monofluorophosphate, all fluoride-releasing compounds form hydrogen fluoride when mixed with hydrochloric acid in the stomach. In the acid environment of the stomach, fluoride and hydrogen ions form the nonionized molecule hydrogen fluoride, which might be irritating to the stomach mucosa if the concentration is sufficiently high. Hydrogen fluoride has been shown to induce structural and functional adverse effects on the gastric mucosa of rats and dogs at concentrations of 190 mg/L. These effects range from loss of the mucous layer and scattered desquamation of mucous cells to widespread erosions of the gastric mucosa (Whitford, 1990).

Experimental studies in rodents given extremely high doses of NaF (1,900 mg/L) demonstrated erosive and hemorrhagic injury to the gastric mucosa and disruption of the structure and integrity of the gastric glands; healing progressed over 7 days (Easmann et al., 1984, 1985; Pashley et al., 1984). In rats, chronic exposure to NaF at 4, 10, or 25 mg/kg in the diet resulted in dose-dependent chronic gastritis and glandular stomach acanthosis (Appendix D in PHS, 1991). Gross lesions were observed in the mucosa of the glandular stomach of male rats treated for 6 months with NaF at 300 mg/L (NTP, 1990). The lesions in male and female rats included diffuse hyperplasia of the mucosal epithelium accompanied by cellular necrosis.

Studies of workers occupationally exposed to varying concentrations of fluoride have reported a variety of gastrointestinal effects. These include chronic gastritis with or without accompanying skeletal fluorosis, duodenal ulcers, and erosion of the gastric mucosa (Medvedeva, 1983; Desai et al., 1986). Neither of the studies reported ambient fluoride measurements, so the actual exposure concentrations are unknown but are presumed to be high.

In summary, high concentrations of fluoride, in the form of hydrogen fluoride, which is due to mixing in the stomach with hydrochloric acid, can be irritating to the gastric mucosa, resulting in dose-dependent adverse effects. There are limited data on humans at low exposures, indicating that at optimal concentrations of fluoride, gastrointestinal effects are not a problem.

HYPERSENSITIVITY AND IMMUNOLOGICAL EFFECTS

Few animal and human data on sodium fluoride-related hyper-sensitivity reactions are found in the literature. In animal studies, ex-cessively high doses, inappropriate routes of administration of fluoride, or both were used (Lewis and Wilson, 1985; Jain and Susheela, 1987). Thus, the predictive value of those data, in relation to human exposures at accepted exposure levels, is questionable. Reports of hypersensitivity reactions in humans resulting from exposure to NaF are mostly anecdotal (Arnold et al., 1960; Richmond, 1985; Modly and Burnett, 1987; Razak and Latifah, 1988). The most common reactions observed included dermatitis, urticaria, inflammation of the oral mucosa, and gastrointestin-al disturbances. Hypersensitivity reactions to fluoride dental preparations were mild to moderately severe and appeared to resolve completely with discontinuation of the product (Adair, 1989). It was reported that those reactions were caused by NaF or by alcohol, dyes, or flavoring agents in the products.

Waldbott (1962) reported that ingestion of fluoride at 1 mg/L of water produced numerous symptoms, which included gastrointestinal distress and joint pains. Those symptoms were also reported in a few patients who received a daily dose of 20 mg or more in treatment for bone conditions (Rich et al., 1964; Shambaugh and Sundar, 1969). However, those symptoms are not believed to be caused by chronic intake of fluoride at any concentration, let alone at the low fluoride concentrations cited by Waldbott. The findings should be disregarded for the following reasons: (1) insufficient clinical and laboratory evidence of allergy or intolerance to fluorides used in the fluoridation of community water, and

(2) no evidence of immunologically mediated reactions in a review of the reported allergic reactions (Austen et al., 1971).

Waldbott (1978) proposed that the skin lesion Chizzola maculae might be caused by airborne fluorides. Waldbott and Cecilioni (1969) attributed the development of these discrete skin lesions to fluoride exposure in 10 of 32 persons living near fertilizer plants in Ontario, Canada, and Iowa and close to an iron foundry in Michigan. Evidence for Chizzola maculae resulting from exposure to fluoride has been reviewed extensively by several investigators (Hodge and Smith, 1977), who concluded that the evidence was circumstantial and unsupported by field surveys.

The literature pertaining to immunological and immunomodulation effects of fluoride is limited. Although direct exposure to high concentrations of NaF in vitro affects a variety of enzymatic activities (Alm, 1983; Mircevova et al., 1984; National Health and Medical Research Council, 1985; Takanaka and O'Brien, 1985; O'Shea et al., 1987; Okada and Brown, 1988; Mizuguchi et al., 1989), the relevance of the effects in vivo is unclear. Standardized immunotoxicity tests of NaF at relevant concentrations and routes of administration have not been conducted.

DISCUSSION

The kidney and gastrointestinal system are exposed to varying fluoride concentrations owing to specific characteristics of fluoride kinetics and excretion patterns. The kidney exhibits the highest tissue-to-plasma fluoride concentrations measured for any soft tissue with a concentration gradient existing across the different anatomic sections of the kidney. All the soluble fluoride-releasing compounds except monophosphate form hydrogen fluoride when mixed with hydrochloric acid in the stomach. Hydrogen fluoride is irritating to the stomach mucosa. For the kidney, experimental studies have demonstrated transient renal effects at relatively high fluoride concentrations (50-100 mg/L). Human epidemiological studies have not observed increased rates of renal disease in populations exposed to fluoride concentrations up to 8 mg/L of drinking water. Experimental studies of the effects of fluoride on the gastrointestinal tract in several animal species have shown dose-dependent adverse effects, such as chronic gastritis and lesions of the stomach mucosa, at doses as low as 190 mg/L. The limited reports on adverse gastrointestinal effects in humans are primarily studies of persons occupationally exposed to unknown concentrations of fluoride. One problem in those studies is that the workers are exposed to a variety of potentially toxic agents, so the contribution of fluoride exposure to risk of adverse effects on the gastrointestinal system is unknown.

Because of the lack of documented adverse effects on the renal and gastrointestinal systems at fluoride concentrations below 8 mg/L of drinking water, no research recommendations are made at this time. The literature pertaining to immunological and immunomodulation effects of fluoride is limited. The weight of evidence shows that fluoride is unlikely to produce hypersensitivity and other immunological effects.

6 GENOTOXICITY OF FLUORIDE

Fluoride has been tested extensively for its genotoxicity. There are a number of published reports on the genotoxicity of fluoride in microbes, cultured mammalian cells, and animals. These data are summarized in Tables 6-1 through 6-6.

IN VITRO GENOTOXICITY TEST SYSTEMS

Microbes

NaF has been tested extensively for its ability to induce gene mutations in Ames *Salmonella typhimurium* reverse mutation assay by standard plate and preincubation tests and in other microbial systems, with and without metabolic activation at concentrations ranging from 0.1 to 4,421 µg/plate (Table 6-1). The results were negative (Litton Bionetics, 1975; Martin et al., 1979; Gocke et al., 1981; Haworth et al., 1983; Arlauskas et al., 1985; Li et al., 1987a; Tong et al., 1988). However, in a suspension assay (a modification of the standard Ames plate test), Nikiforova (1982) reported positive findings in *S. typhimurium* strains TA1535 and TA98 at concentrations of 1,000-1,500 µg/plate. The reported increases in histidine-revertants (mutations) in *S. typhimurium* strains TA1535 and TA98 appear to be artifactual results of increased cell killing, which

TABLE 6-1 In Vitro Mutagenicity of Fluoride

System	End Point	Exposure Time	Fluoride Exposure	Result	Reference
Salmonella	His reversion	—	0.1-2,000 μg/plate	Negative	Martin et al., 1979
Salmonella	His reversion	—	1,000-1,500 μg/plate	Positive	Nikiforova, 1982
Salmonella	His reversion	—	0.44-4,421 μg/plate	Negative	Li et al., 1987a
Salmonella	His reversion	—	10-320 μg/plate	Negative	Tong et al., 1988
Salmonella	His reversion	—	2-6 μmol/plate	Negative	Gocke et al., 1981
Salmonella	His reversion	—	0.0185-0.074%	Negative	Litton Bionetics, 1975
Saccharomyces cerevisiae D4	Tryp reversion	4 hr	0.00325-0.013%	Negative	Litton Bionetics, 1975
Mouse lymphoma L5178Y	TK, Oua, 6-TG, excess thymidine, methotrexate, Ara C	4, 16, 48 hr	10-500 μg/mL	Positive at all loci except Oua	Cole et al., 1986
Mouse lymphoma L5178Y	TK	4 hr	300-600 μg/mL	Positive	Caspary et al., 1987
Human lymphoblastoid cells	TK	4 hr	200-600 μg/mL	Positive	Caspary et al., 1988
Rat liver epithelial cells	HGPRT	72 hr	2-40 μg/mL	Negative	Tong et al., 1988

Human lympho-blastoid cells	HGPRT	28 hr	200-600 µg/mL	Positive	Crespi et al., 1990
	TK	28 hr	200-600 µg/mL	Positive	
	TK	20 d	65 µg/mL	Positive	
Chinese hamster ovary V79 cells	6-TG resistance	24 hr	10-400 µg/mL	Negative	Slamenová et al., 1992

His = histidine.
TK = thymidine kinase.
Oua = ouabain.
HGPRT = hypoxanthine guanine phosphoribosyl transferase.
Ara C = 1-β-D-arabinofuranosyl cytosine.
Tryp = tryptophan.
6-TG = 6-thioguanine.

might have increased histidine and generated small background colonies. NaF was not mutagenic to *Saccharomyces cerevisiae* strain D4 (Litton Bionetics, 1975). Table 6-1 summarizes mutagenicity data of fluoride in microbial organisms and mammalian cells in culture. NaF was found to be negative in the *Bacillus subtilis* rec assay (Matsui, 1980), a test that measures DNA damage. However, Kanematsu (1985) reported that both NaF and stannous fluoride (SnF_2) were positive. The differing results could be due to the differing protocols used by the two investigators. NaF failed to induce gene conversion and aneuploidy in *S. cerevisiae* (Litton Bionetics, 1975; Martin et al., 1979); similar results were reported for potassium fluoride (KF) when tested in *Neurospora* (Griffiths, 1981).

Mammalian Cells

Fluoride has been tested in in vitro mammalian cell cultures for its ability to induce mutations, chromosomal aberrations, sister chromatid exchanges, DNA damage and repair, and cell transformation.

Gene Mutations

Fluoride has been tested for its mutagenicity in several in vitro mammalian cell systems with and without metabolic activation (Table 6-1). NaF and KF were strongly mutagenic in the mouse lymphoma L5178Y $TK^{+/-}$ test with and without S9 at concentrations ranging from 10 to 600 μg/mL (Cole et al., 1986; Caspary et al., 1987); the authors speculated that the induced mutant colonies resulted from chromosomal damage rather than point (gene) mutations. This hypothesis was supported by the absence of induction of ouabain-resistant mutants in the same cell type (Cole et al., 1986). Caspary et al. (1988) reported that NaF was mutagenic at the *tk* locus in human lymphoblastoid cells treated with NaF at 200-600 μg/mL for 4 hours. Recently, Crespi et al. (1990) reported that NaF was mutagenic at the *tk* and *hgprt* loci in human lymphoblastoid cells treated with NaF at concentrations of 200-600 μg/mL for 28 hours and at the *tk* locus in cells treated with 65 μg/mL for 20 days. However, a statistically significant response was observed only at concentrations that resulted in substantial cell death. In contrast, no mutagenicity was observed at the *hgprt* locus in rat liver epithelial cells treated with NaF at concentrations of 2-40 μg/mL for 72 hours (Tong et al., 1988) or at the 6-*tg* locus in Chinese hamster ovary V79 cells treated with NaF at 10-400 μg/mL for 24 hours (Slamenová et al., 1992).

Chromosomal Aberrations and Sister Chromatid Exchanges

NaF has been shown to induce chromosomal damage in several in vitro mammalian cell systems (Table 6-2). The reported chromosomal effects were primarily chromatid deletions or achromatic lesions (gaps); the definition and scoring of the latter events is not standardized, and their significance is unknown, and, in fact, questionable. These effects were not always clearly demonstrated and appeared to be protocol-dependent (Li et al., 1988; Aardema et al., 1989).

Animal Cells   Chromosomal aberrations were increased by 3 hours of exposure to NaF at concentrations of 25-100 μg/mL in Chinese hamster ovary cells (but not at concentrations of 0.1-10 μg/mL) (Aardema et al., 1989), at 50-200 μg/mL in Syrian hamster embryo cells (Tsutsui et al., 1984a), and at 12.6-126 μg/mL in red muntjac cells (He et al., 1983). Aardema et al. (1989) concluded that the G2 stage of the cell cycle is a sensitive stage for NaF-induced chromosomal damage in Chinese hamster ovary cells. Chromosomal abnormalities also were reported in Chinese hamster ovary Don cells treated with NaF at 25-75 μg/mL for 12-36 hours (Bale and Mathew, 1987). The National Toxicology Program studies (NTP, 1990) in Chinese hamster ovary cells showed no induction of aberrations in one laboratory where NaF was tested at concentrations up to 200 μg/mL without S9 and harvested after 20½ hours, but a positive response was reported in a second laboratory at concentrations of 400-600 μg/mL with a shorter (13 hours) harvest time. No chromosomal aberrations were induced with metabolic activation at concentrations up to 1,600 μg/mL at either harvest time (NTP, 1990). No chromosomal aberrations were induced in Chinese hamster lung cells by NaF at concentrations up to 500 μg/mL (Ishidate, 1988).

TABLE 6-2 Cytogenetic Effects of Fluoride in Cultured Mammalian Cells

System	End Point	Exposure Time, hr	Fluoride, µg/mL	Result	Reference
Animal Cells					
Chinese hamster ovary cells	Aberrations	3	0.1-1,276	Positive	Aardema et al., 1989
Syrian hamster ovary cells	Aberrations	16, 28	50-200	Positive	Tsutsui et al., 1984a
Syrian hamster ovary cells	SCE	24	20-80	Positive	Tsutsui et al., 1984a
Red muntjac	SCE	—	12.6-126	Positive	He et al., 1983
Red muntjac	Aberrations	—	12.6-126	Positive	He et al., 1983
Chinese hamster ovary Don cells	Aberrations	12, 24, 36	25-75	Positive	Bale and Matthew, 1987
Chinese hamster ovary cells	Aberrations	—	1.6-1,600	Positive	NTP, 1990
Chinese hamster ovary cells	SCE	—	1.6-1,600	Positive	NTP, 1990
Chinese hamster ovary cells	SCE	24	2-160	Negative	Tong et al., 1988
Human Cells					
Lymphocytes	Aberrations	2	20-40	Positive	Albanese, 1987
Fibroblasts	Aberrations	24-72	10-20	Positive	Scott and Roberts, 1987
Fibroblasts	Aberrations	12-24	20-75	Positive	Tsutsui et al., 1984b

Leukocytes	Aberrations	24	1-132	Positive	Jachimczak and Skotarczak, 1978
Lymphocytes	Aberrations	24	11-44	Positive	Sato et al., 1989
Lymphocytes	Aberrations	2	46-130	Negative	Voroshilin et al., 1973
Lymphocytes	Aberrations	24-72	0.25-10	Negative	Kralisz and Saymaniak, 1978
Lymphocytes	Aberrations	24	1-16	Negative	Matsuda, 1980
Lymphocytes	Aberrations	2	4.2-42	Negative	Gebhart et al., 1984
Lymphocytes	SCE	48	4.2-580	Negative	Thomson et al., 1985
Lymphocytes	SCE	48	2-80	Negative	Tong et al., 1988

SCE = Sister chromatid exchanges.

Sister chromatid exchanges were not induced by NaF in Chinese hamster ovary cells treated with 250 μg/mL for 24 hours (Li et al., 1987b) or with 160 μg/mL for 24 hours (Tong et al., 1988). However, sister chromatid exchanges were induced in Syrian hamster embryo cells treated with 20-80 μg/mL without S9 (Tsutsui et al., 1984a), and in red muntjac cells treated with 126 μg/mL (He et al., 1983). In the NTP studies, the incidence of sister chromatid exchanges was increased in Chinese hamster ovary cells treated with NaF at concentrations up to 1,600 μg/mL with S9.

Human Cells   Several investigators have reported chromosomal aberrations in cultured human lymphocytes and fibroblasts at NaF concentrations ranging from 20 to 40 μg/mL (Tsutsui, et al., 1984b; Albanese, 1987; Scott and Roberts, 1987). Chromosomal aberrations were also observed in human leukocytes at concentrations ranging from 1 to 132 μg/mL (Jachimczak and Skotarczak, 1978). Sato et al. (1989) reported the induction of chromosomal gaps, but not breaks or rearrangements, in human lymphocytes treated with fluoride at concentrations up to 44 μg/mL. However, other investigators did not observe chromosomal aberrations in human lymphocytes and leukocytes exposed in vitro to NaF at concentrations up to 125 μg/mL (Voroshilin et al., 1975; Kralisz and Szymaniak, 1978; Matsuda, 1980; Gebhart et al., 1984). Sister chromatid exchanges were also not observed in human lymphocytes exposed to NaF at concentrations up to 420 μg/mL or KF at concentrations up to 580 μg/mL (Thomson et al., 1985; Tong et al., 1988).

DNA Damage and Repair

Several investigators have studied the induction of DNA repair synthesis and unscheduled DNA synthesis in various in vitro mammalian cell systems (Table 6-3). NaF has been shown to inhibit protein and DNA synthesis in cultured mammalian cells (Holland, 1979a,b; Li et al., 1988); the inhibition of DNA synthesis might be a secondary effect of the inhibition of protein synthesis or a direct inhibition of DNA polymerase (Skare et al., 1986a; Holland 1979a,b; Imai et al., 1983). NaF failed to induce DNA repair synthesis in primary rat hepatocytes at concentrations up to 160 μg/mL (Tong et al., 1988). Skare et al. (1986a) did not

TABLE 6-3 Effect of Fluoride Exposure on Induction of DNA
Repair Synthesis and Unscheduled DNA Synthesis

System	Exposure Time, hr	Flouride, μg/mL	Result	Reference
DNA repair synthesis in rat hepatocytes	18	2-160	Negative	Tong et al., 1988
UDS in human fibroblasts	1.5-8	8-500	Negative	Skare et al., 1986a
UDS in rat hepatocytes	18-20	8-120	Negative	Skare et al., 1986a
UDS in Syrian hamster embryo cells	12	10-40	Positive	Tsutsui et al., 1984a
UDS in human oral keratinocytes	4	100-300	Positive	Tsutsui et al., 1984c

UDS = Unscheduled DNA synthesis.

observe unscheduled DNA synthesis in human fibroblasts treated with
NaF at 8-500 μg/mL. NaF at concentrations of 10-300 μg/mL induced
unscheduled DNA synthesis in Syrian hamster cells (Tsutsui et al.,
1984a) and in human keratinocytes (Tsutsui et al., 1984c), but those
results were not confirmed by other investigators who used concentrations
that did not induce high levels of toxicity (Skare et al., 1986a; Tong et
al., 1988).

Transformation

Transformation is a process that changes a normal cell into one that is
capable of forming a tumor that might or might not be malignant. The
main event that initiates transformation is a change in the genetic material.

Several investigators have studied the ability of NaF to transform cells
in culture (see Table 6-4). Dose-related increases in the frequencies of
transformed colonies were observed in Syrian hamster embryo cells at
NaF concentrations of 10-125 μg/mL (Tsutsui et al., 1984a; Jones et al.,
1988a,b; Lasne et al., 1988). Morphological transformation was not
induced in BALB/3T3 cells treated with NaF for 72 hours at concentra-

TABLE 6-4   Effect of Fluoride on Cell Transformation

System	End Point	Exposure Time, d	Fluoride, μg/mL	Result	Reference
Syrian hamster embryo cells	Morphological transformation	1	75-125	Positive	Tsutsui et al., 1984a
Syrian hamster embryo cells	Neoplastic transformation	1	75-100	Positive	Tsutsui et al., 1984a
Syrian hamster embryo cells	Morphological transformation	4	10-50	Positive	Jones et al., 1988a
Syrian hamster embryo cells	Morphological transformation	7	25-125	Positive	Jones et al., 1988b
Syrian hamster embryo cells	Morphological transformation	7	75-125	Positive	Lasne et al., 1988
BALB/3T3 cells	Foci	3	25-50	Negative[a] Positive[b]	Lasne et al., 1988

[a] In standard assay.
[b] In "promotion"-type assay.

tions of 25-50 μg/mL (Lasne et al., 1988). Syrian hamster embryo cells transformed by NaF at 75 or 100 μg/mL and injected into newborn Syrian hamsters produced tumors at the site of injection after 141-320 days (Tsutsui et al., 1984a). Histological examination of the tumors formed in vivo revealed that the tumors were anaplastic fibrosarcomas.

It should be noted that hamster embryo cells are unusually sensitive to the induction of transformation and are not considered to be representative of the transformation susceptibility of other cell types. Thus, the overall significance of the fluoride transformation data are subject to question.

Discussion

If there is a threshold concentration of fluoride for genotoxicity in in vitro tests, how does it compare with concentrations found in humans? The results of mammalian-cell culture studies show a lowest effective dose at approximately 10 μg/mL (NaF at 10 μg is equivalent to fluoride ion at 4.5 μg). That concentration should be compared with the steady-state concentration of fluoride ion at 0.02-0.06 μg/mL in human plasma that exists even in areas where water supplies are fluoridated. If it is accepted that the sensitivity of human fibroblasts in vitro is a fair representation of cellular sensitivity in vivo and if a true threshold does exist, then clearly there is a large safety margin (Scott and Roberts, 1987).

IN VIVO GENOTOXICITY TEST SYSTEMS

NaF and other fluoride salts have been tested for their genotoxicity in *Drosophila* and rodents. As shown above in the in vitro test results, the in vivo test results are also mixed. The published data are generally weak and the descriptions of experimental protocols often fail to provide dose-selection criteria and toxicity information, thus precluding accurate assessment of the adequacy of the test concentrations.

Drosophila

Several reports on the genotoxicity of NaF and other fluoride-containing compounds in *Drosophila* have been published (Table 6-5). Most of the studies used inadequate controls, thereby preventing assessment of the effect of NaF alone. However, there are a few studies that allow critical analyses of the mutagenicity of fluoride. Gerdes (1971) exposed *Drosophila* males to hydrogen fluoride (HF) at 2.9 ppm and 4.3 ppm by inhalation and observed dose-related increases in sex-linked recessive lethal mutations. Similar results were obtained by Mitchell and Gerdes (1973) when NaF and SnF_2 were administered to *Drosophila* by feeding in a glucose solution. Vogel (1973) reported that NaF in diet induced whole chromosomal loss and partial chromosomal loss, an indication of chromosomal breakage in postmeiotic germ cells of males. However, Gocke et al. (1981) reported that feeding of SnF_2 or sodium monofluorophosphate (Na_2FPO_3) did not induce sex-linked recessive lethal mutations in *Drosophila*. Other studies have reported no induction of sex-linked recessive lethal mutations (Mukherjee and Sobels, 1968; MacDonald and Luker, 1980) or dominant lethality and sex-chromosome loss (Büchi and Bürki, 1975), but the genetic systems used or the numbers of flies treated or examined probably were inadequate.

TABLE 6-5 In Vivo Mutation Effects of Fluoride in *Drosophila*

End Point	Route	Exposure Time	Fluoride Dose	Result	Reference
Sex-linked recessive lethal	—	—	2.9-4.3 ppm	Positive	Gerdes, 1971
Sex-linked recessive lethal	Diet	—	—	Positive	Mitchell and Gerdes, 1973
Sex-chromosome loss	Diet	17 hr	228 ppm	Positive	Vogel, 1973
Sperm fertility	Diet	17 hr	46-456 ppm	Negative	Vogel, 1973
Recessive lethal, sex-chromosome loss, nondisjunction	Diet	3 d	91,228 ppm	Negative, positive, negative	Vogel, 1973
Sex-linked recessive lethal	Diet	—	1.25-2.5 mM[a]	Negative	Gocke et al., 1981
Sex-linked recessive lethal	Diet	—	228 ppm	Negative	MacDonald and Luker, 1980
Sex-chromosome loss, dominant lethal	Diet	—	385 ppm	Negative	Büchi and Bürki, 1975
Recovery of sex-chromosome loss, chromosome translocation	Diet	—	112.5 ppm	Negative	Mendelson, 1976
Sex-linked recessive lethal	—	—	190 ppm	Negative	Mukherjee and Sobels, 1968

[a]mM = millimolar.

Rodents

Fluoride has been tested for its in vivo genotoxicity in mice, rats, and hamsters. The in vivo studies in rodents include tests for mutations, chromosomal aberrations, sister chromatid exchanges, DNA damage, and related genotoxic effects in germ cells (Table 6-6).

Somatic Cells

Induction of sister chromatid exchanges, chromosomal aberrations, and micronuclei was reported in the bone-marrow cells of mice administered NaF at 10-40 mg/kg of body weight by gavage and by intraperitoneal or subcutaneous injection (Ma et al., 1986; Pati and Bhunya, 1987). However, the study of Ma et al. (1986) is presented in abstract form and no data are available; Pati and Bhunya (1987) included chromatid gaps and breaks in their analysis of aberrations and relied largely on the gaps for their conclusions that NaF was clastogenic. The results were dose- and time-dependent but showed no route sensitivity. Fractionated dosing yielded weaker genotoxic response. The significance of gaps is not understood, and they are not normally used in aberration analysis. In contrast, no clastogenic effects were seen in bone marrow of Swiss-Webster mice administered NaF at 50 mg/kg in feed for seven generations (Kram et al., 1978). Martin et al. (1979) also did not observe increased frequency of chromosomal aberrations in bone marrow or testis cells of Swiss-Webster mice that received fluoride at either 50 mg/L for at least five generations or 1-100 mg/L for 6 months as compared with animals that received distilled water.

Mohamed and Chandler (1982) administered drinking water containing fluoride at 0, 1, 5, 10, 50, 100, or 200 mg/L to BALB/c mice for 3-6 weeks. Cytological studies on bone-marrow-cell chromosomes showed that NaF at 1-200 mg/L induced chromosomal changes in a dose-dependent manner. The frequency of the induced chromosomal damage was significantly higher at fluoride concentrations as little as 1 mg/L. However, because of the very high frequency of aberrant cells in control animals and uncertainty regarding the nature of aberrations scored, the validity of these findings is questionable. Li et al. (1989) conducted a

TABLE 6-6 In Vivo Chromosome Effects of Fluoride

System	End Point	Route	Exposure Time	Fluoride Dose	Result	Reference
BALB/c mice	Aberrations	Water	3-6 wk	1-200 mg/L	Positive	Mohamed and Chandler, 1982
Swiss-Webster mice	Sister chromatid exchanges	Diet	7 generations	<0.5, 50 mg/kg	Negative	Kram et al., 1978
Swiss-Webster mice	Aberrations in bone-marrow cells	Water	5 generations (2 yr)	50 mg/L	Negative	Martin et al., 1979
Swiss-Webster mice	Aberrations in bone-marrow cells	Water	6 wk	1-100 mg/L	Negative	Martin et al., 1979
B6C3F$_1$ mice	Micronucleus	Gavage	Acute	0.1-115 mg/kg	Negative	Li et al., 1987
Swiss mice	Aberrations	i.p. Gavage s.c.	Acute Acute Acute	10-40 mg/kg 10-40 mg/kg 10-40 mg/kg	Positive Positive Positive	Pati and Bhunya, 1987
Swiss mice	Micronucleus	i.p.	3 doses, 24 hr apart	10-40 mg/kg	Positive	Pati and Bhunya, 1987
Mice	Micronucleus	i.p.	Acute	7.5-30 (NaF) 20-80 (Na$_2$FPO$_3$) mg/kg	Negative	Hayashi et al., 1988
White mice	Aberrations	Inhalation	6 hr/d, 6 d/wk for 2 mo	0.1 mg/m^3	Negative	Voroshilin et al., 1975
NMRI mice	Micronucleus	i.p.	2 doses in 24 hr	9.8-39.5 mg/kg	Negative	Gocke et al., 1981
BALB/c mice	Micronucleus	Water	21 wk	1-75 mg/L	Negative	Dunipace et al., 1989
Swiss mice	Sister chromatid exchanges	i.p.	2 doses, acute	7, 20 mg/kg	Positive	Ma et al., 1986

Species/strain	Endpoint	Route	Duration	Dose	Result	Reference
Swiss mice	Micronucleus	Gavage	2 doses, 24 hr apart	20 mg/kg	Positive	Ma et al., 1986
AP rats	Micronucleus	Gavage	Acute	500-1,000 mg/kg	Negative	Albanese, 1987
Chinese hamsters	Sister chromatid exchanges	Water	21 wk	1-75 mg/L	Negative	Li et al., 1989
Sprague-Dawley rats	DNA-strand breaks in testis	Gavage	5 d	8.4-84 mg/kg	Negative	Skare et al., 1986b
B6C3F$_1$ mice	Sperm head abnormality	Water	21 wk	1-75 mg/L	Negative	Dunipace et al., 1989
Swiss mice	Sperm abnormality	i.p.	5 daily	10-40 mg/kg	Positive	Pati and Bhunya, 1987
Swiss-Webster mice	Aberrations in testis cells	Water	5 generations (2 yr)	50 mg/L	Negative	Martin et al., 1979
B6C3F$_1$ mice	Sperm head abnormality	Gavage	5 d	0.1-70 mg/kg	Negative	Li et al., 1987d
BALB/c mice	Aberrations in spermatocytes	Water	3 or 6 wk	1-200 mg/L	Positive	Mohamed and Chandler, 1982

i.p. = intraperitoneal.
s.c. = subcutaneous.

bone-marrow sister-chromatid-exchange study in which NaF at 1, 10, 50, or 75 mg/L of drinking water was administered to male Chinese hamsters for 21 weeks. No significant increases in sister chromatid exchanges were observed, even though fluoride concentrations in bone and plasma increased with NaF treatment.

Micronuclei contain one (usually) or several chromosomes or chromosome fragments that are not included in the nuclei formed at mitotic cell division. They persist in one of the daughter cells for only one or several subsequent divisions. Thus, micronuclei represent loss of genetic material from a body cell (as opposed to reproductive cells: sperm and eggs), which eventually leads to the death of that cell. Because micronuclei are scored at the long interphase stage of the cell cycle, they serve as a rapid screen for agents that interfere with normal mitotic chromosome and cell division.

Micronuclei were not induced in the bone marrow of mice injected once intraperitoneally with NaF at 30 mg/kg or Na_2FPO_3 at 80 mg/kg (Hayashi et al., 1988) or injected twice with SnF_2 at up to 39.5 mg/kg (Gocke et al., 1981). When Li and co-workers (1987c) administered NaF by gavage to male and female B6C3F$_1$ mice in doses up to the maximum tolerated dose (MTD) (80 mg/kg for males and 115 mg/kg for females), the mice did not show increased micronucleated polychromatic erythrocytes in their bone marrow. Pati and Bhunya (1987) reported increases in micronuclei in bone marrow polychromatic erythrocytes of Swiss mice that received two intraperitoneal injections of NaF at 10-40 mg/kg. No micronuclei were induced in the bone marrow of male AP rats that received NaF at 500 or 1,000 mg/kg by gavage (Albanese, 1987). Dunipace et al. (1989) did not observe micronuclei in polychromatic erythrocytes of B6C3F$_1$ mice that were given NaF in drinking water at concentrations of 1-75 mg/L for 21 weeks.

Germ Cells

In the Mohamed and Chandler (1982) study in which BALB/c mice were given drinking water containing fluoride at 0, 1, 5, 10, 50, 100, or 200 mg/L for 3-6 weeks, cytological tests showed that NaF at 1-200 mg/L induced chromosomal aberrations in spermatocytes in a dose-dependent manner. However, Martin et al. (1979) did not observe chromosomal aberrations in mitotic or meiotic cells of testes of mice that were administered fluoride at 1-100 mg/L of drinking water for 6 weeks or maintained for several generations on 50 mg/L of drinking water. Inhalation of HF at 0.1 mg/m^3, 6 hours per day, 6 days per week for 2-4 weeks did not induce aberrations in meiotic chromosomes of the testes of white mice (Voroshilin et al., 1975). Dominant lethal mutations were not observed in male white mice that inhaled HF at concentrations of 1 mg/m^3 for 2-4 weeks (Voroshilin et al., 1975). A study on sperm-head morphology in Swiss mice exposed intraperitoneally to NaF at 10-40 mg/kg for 5 days and then sampled 35 days later reported a large dose-dependent increase in abnormal sperm (Pati and Bhunya, 1987). However, no morphological abnormalities were observed in sperm from mice that drank water containing fluoride at concentrations of 75 g/L for 21 weeks (Dunipace et al., 1989) or that were given fluoride at up to 70 mg/kg by gavage for 5 days (Li et al., 1987d). No DNA single-strand breaks were observed in testicular cells of rats that were administered NaF by gavage at up to 84 mg/kg per day for 5 days (Skare et al., 1986b). Genotoxicity of fluoride in germ cells of mammals cannot be evaluated because of insufficient data.

Human Studies

There are no published studies in the literature on the genetic or cytogenetic effects of fluoride in humans.

PROPOSED MECHANISMS OF GENOTOXICITY

The mechanism of genotoxicity of fluoride is not known. A number of possible mechanisms have been postulated to explain the observed genotoxicity of fluoride (NTP, 1990; PHS, 1991). Fluoride is not a typical mutagen. It cannot intercalate (invade and insert) into the DNA molecule and therefore cannot form DNA adducts, which can result in mutation. Furthermore, the results of many studies conducted to determine the genotoxicity of fluoride often conflict, making it difficult to explain the mechanisms of genotoxicity of fluoride. Nonetheless, clues to how fluoride affects genetic integrity can be found in the interaction of fluoride with cellular components. Speculations on mechanisms of genetic toxicity have been based on the observed reactions of fluoride in solution with divalent cations or nucleotides or the physiological and biochemical responses of cells treated with fluoride. NaF inhibits protein and DNA synthesis in cultured mammalian cells (Holland, 1979a). The inhibition of DNA synthesis might be a secondary effect of the inhibition of protein synthesis or a direct effect of the inhibition of DNA polymerase or other DNA synthesis-associated enzymes. Fluoride can react with divalent cations in the cell to affect enzyme activities that are necessary for DNA or RNA synthesis or chromosomal metabolism or maintenance; it might react directly with DNA as part of a complex; or it can disrupt other cellular processes, such as cell differentiation or energy metabolism (Hellung-Larsen and Klenow, 1969; Harper et al., 1974; Holland, 1979a,b; Srivastava et al., 1981; Imai et al., 1983; Edwards and Parry, 1986). A hypothesis of secondary effects on DNA or chromosomes is attractive because there is no apparent mechanism by which many of the genotoxic effects observed can be induced by direct interaction of fluoride with DNA.

SUMMARY

The in vitro data indicate that (1) the genotoxicity of fluoride is limited primarily to doses much higher than those to which humans are exposed, (2) even at high doses, genotoxic effects are not always observed, and (3) the preponderance of the genotoxic effects that have been reported are of the types that probably are of no or negligible genetic significance.

In vivo tests in rodents for genotoxicity of fluoride provide mixed results that cannot be resolved readily because of differences in protocols and insufficient detail in some reports to allow a thorough analysis.

7 CARCINOGENICITY OF FLUORIDE

FLUORIDE CARCINOGENICITY IN HUMANS

More than 50 epidemiological studies have evaluated the possibility of an association between fluoride concentrations in drinking water and human cancer. With one exception, the available studies are geographic correlation studies or geographic time-trend correlation studies in which measures of exposure and disease are made at the community level. The strengths and limitations of such ecological studies are addressed in Chapter 3.

Because of the continuing importance of the question of fluoride in drinking water and human cancer, the relevant scientific literature has been exhaustively reviewed by several independent expert panels of epidemiologists. The two most comprehensive evaluations were conducted by the British Working Party on the Fluoridation of Water and Cancer under the chairmanship of E.G. Knox (Knox, 1985) and by an international panel of epidemiologists convened by the Monographs Programme of the International Agency for Research on Cancer in Lyon, France (IARC, 1982). In addition, the epidemiological literature was reviewed by a subcommittee of the Drinking Water Committee of the National Research Council (NRC, 1977). The latter review was less detailed than the Knox and IARC reports but reached similar conclusions; it will not be considered further here. The Knox and IARC panels considered all the available evidence relating to fluoride in drinking water and cancer in human populations. Given the high quality of the critical literature reviews already completed by Knox and co-workers, IARC, and other groups, the subcommittee elected to briefly summarize their findings and conclusions rather than conduct another independent review of the available literature. There have been few contributions to the literature since the publication of the Knox report (Knox, 1985). Eight studies deserve consideration (Lynch, 1984; Hrudey et al., 1990; Hoover et al., 1991a,b; McGuire et al., 1991; Mahoney et al., 1991; Cohn, 1992; Freni and Gaylor, 1992). They will be described and evaluated separately.

As noted earlier, correlations of exposure and disease or mortality rates among population aggregations made in ecological studies are subject to certain limitations. However, the exposure measure used in correlational studies of fluoridated water and cancer is unusual in that it applies to most or all individuals within a study area. Therefore, such studies might be better indicators of risk than other correlational studies, such as occupational or ethnicity studies, in which only a small fraction of a country's population usually is truly exposed. All the expert panels noted the relative strengths and weaknesses of the correlation studies.

The expert panel reviews generally agree that available data provide no credible evidence for an association between either naturally occurring fluoride or added fluoride in drinking water and risk of human cancer. A series of studies begun in 1975 by Yiamouyiannis and colleagues showed both geographic and temporal associations between fluoride in drinking water and risk of cancer mortality (e.g., Yiamouyiannis and Burk, 1977). However, as revealed in great detail in Chapters 3 and 4 of the Knox report (Knox, 1985) and in many other critiques, those studies did not adjust adequately for differences in age, race, and sex of the compared populations. That resulted in inappropriate comparisons of groups that differed in one or more of those demographic factors. The Knox report concluded that there is "no reliable evidence of any hazard to man in respect to cancer." The IARC group (1982) came to a similar conclusion, namely, that "Variations geographically and in time in the fluoride content of water supplies provide no evidence of an association between fluoride ingestion and mortality from cancer in humans." The panels that evaluated the available epidemiological data on fluoride in drinking water recognized the limitations of demographic correlational studies in providing fully adequate data to make such evaluations. Lynch (1984) conducted a study using cancer incidence in Iowa municipalities for the years 1969-1981. The relation between cancer incidence and added or natural fluoride in drinking water was analyzed in 158 municipalities with a total 1970 population of 1,414,878. A total of 66,572 cancer cases (comprising cancer of all sites, the bladder, female breast, colon, lung, prostate, rectum, and other sites combined) were evaluated in four study groups, two each for added fluoride and for natural fluoride. In addition, the duration of exposure to fluoridated water was evaluated. Univariate and multivariate cancer-site, sex-specific statistical analyses were performed. Eight sociodemographic variables were evaluated in multivariate models to account for any effect they might have had on the fluoride-cancer relation. The results showed inconsistent relations between the fluoride variable and cancer incidence and failed to support a fluoride-cancer association.

Hoover et al. (1991a) updated an earlier analysis of cancer mortality by county in the United States (Hoover et al., 1976) as related to county drinking-water fluoridation. The analysis used records of over 2,208,000 cancer deaths by county for 1950-1985 to examine possible changes in county cancer mortality over that period. The study was restricted to the white population to avoid confounding by racial variations in cancer mortality rates. Comparisons of age-adjusted cancer mortality by anatomic site and sex were made between fluoridated and nonfluoridated counties for time periods preceding and following fluoridation. Cancers of the bones and joints (osteosarcoma is not reported separately in mortality statistics) were singled out for detailed analysis because of results of animal studies. Among both males and females residing in counties with rapid fluoridation (at least two-thirds of the population receiving fluoridated water within 3 years), the risk of death from cancers of bones and joints 20-35 years after fluoridation was the same as it was in the years immediately preceding fluoridation. Cancer-incidence data, as related to fluoridation status of drinking water, were also analyzed in counties of two geographic regions covered by the Surveillance, Epidemiology and End Results Program (SEER), a large tumor registry supported by the National Cancer Institute. Both regions comprised fluoridated and nonfluoridated counties. Over 125,000 newly diagnosed cases were included. For all types of malignancy, there was no evidence of a consistent relation between cancer incidence or mortality and patterns of fluoridation. An additional study of cancer incidence in SEER areas analyzed incidence rates of osteosarcoma as well as all bone and joint cancers with respect to time of fluoridation (Hoover et al., 1992b). Although the rates of osteosarcoma were generally higher in the fluoridated areas than in the nonfluoridated areas, they bore no relation to time of fluoridation.

McGuire et al. (1991) conducted a small case-control study of osteosarcoma that included telephone interviews with 22 patients and matched controls. No association was found between osteosarcoma and average lifetime or childhood exposure to fluoride in drinking water. The small size of the population restricted the statistical power of this study to detect associations.

A study of cancer-incidence rates in fluoridated and nonfluoridated communities in New York conducted by Mahoney et al. (1991) evaluated time trends of all bone-cancer rates between 1950 and 1987 and time trends of osteosarcoma rates between 1970 and 1987; a comparison of bone-cancer and osteosarcoma rates among males and females between 1976 and 1987 was also performed. Total bone cancer increased significantly in males less than 30 years of age, amounting to a 54% increase between 1955 and 1987, but decreased significantly in males and females (separately) 30 years of age and older. Osteosarcoma did not increase significantly in males of either age group or in females. The average annual sex- and age-specific rates of bone cancer and osteosarcoma for 1970-1987 did not differ in areas with or without fluoridated drinking water.

An ecological study in seven central New Jersey counties observed a higher rate of osteosarcoma in fluoridated communities than in nonfluoridated communities in 1979-1987 (a risk ratio of 3.4 among males under 20 years of age) (Cohn, 1992). Osteosarcoma was diagnosed in 12 males under 20 years of age in fluoridated communities versus eight males in nonfluoridated communities. Rate ratios comparing fluoridated with nonfluoridated communities were not elevated among females or among males in older age groups. The question of osteosarcoma rates in young males with respect to time of fluoridation was not examined in this study.

A study in the Province of Alberta, Canada, compared the annual incidence rates of osteosarcoma for 1970-1988 in Edmonton, where water was first fluoridated in 1967, with rates in Calgary, where water was fluoridated in the fall of 1989 (Hrudey et al., 1990). The data showed no difference in rates between the municipalities and showed no time trend. The average annual incidence rates for 1970-1988 were 0.27 per 100,000 in Edmonton and 0.29 per 100,000 in Calgary, based on 26 and 29 cases, respectively.

Freni and Gaylor (1992) conducted a time-trend analysis of bone-cancer incidence in the United States, Canada, and Europe. Bone-cancer incidence rates were obtained from 40 cancer registries covering a population of 150 million people for periods of 3-6 years spanning the period 1958-1987. A registry area was considered fluoridated if fluoride at approximately 1 mg/L was added to the drinking water of a least 50% of the registry population in the 1960s or before. Because bone cancer is rare, the cumulative risk among people 10-29 years of age or 0-74 years of age was used to examine time trends. Significant increases in the cumulative risk of bone cancer were noted primarily among young males in some registry areas in the United States; significant decreases in lifetime risk were noted among both sexes in Europe. Neither the American increase nor the European decrease in risk was related to fluoridation.

Findings from the additional studies support the conclusions of the Knox report and the IARC panel in that they provide no credible evidence for an association between fluoride in drinking water and risk of cancer.

FLUORIDE CARCINOGENICITY IN ANIMALS

The subcommittee reviewed six carcinogenicity studies in animals that have been reported in the literature to date (Table 7-1). However, only two carcinogenicity studies conducted by NTP and Procter & Gamble are considered adequate for determining the carcinogenic activity in animals. The first four studies are inadequate because of deficiencies in design or documentation of results, although they were consistently negative for an association of fluoride with carcinogenicity.

Early Toxicological Studies Of Fluoride and Cancer

Tannenbaum and Silverstone (1949) showed that the addition of 0.09% (10 mg/kg of body weight) sodium fluoride to the diets of female mice

TABLE 7-1 Studies of Fluoride Carcinogenicity in Animals

Study	Sex/Species	Route	Dose	Results
Tannenbaum and Silverstone, 1949	Female mice	Diet	10 mg/kg	Negative
Taylor, 1954	Female mice	Drinking water	0.4-10 mg/L	Negative
Taylor and Taylor, 1965	Mice[a]	Drinking water	1-5 mg/L	Accelerated growth of mammary gland
Kanisawa and Schroeder, 1969	Male and female mice	Drinking water	10 mg/L	Negative
NTP study (Bucher et al., 1991)	Male rats	Drinking water	25, 100, 175 mg/L	Equivocal increase in osteosarcomas
NTP study (Bucher et al., 1991)	Female rats, and male and female mice	Drinking water	25, 100, 175 mg/L	Negative
P&G study (Maurer et al., 1990)	Male and female rats	Diet	4, 10, 25 mg/kg	Negative
P&G study (Maurer et al., in press)	Male and female mice	Diet	4, 10, 25 mg/kg	Observation of osteomas

[a]Sex not specified.

resulted in a 10-40% reduction in body weight without a reduction in caloric intake. Mice on the fluoride diets also drank notably more water than did controls. There was a marked reduction in the incidence of spontaneous mammary tumors: after 100 weeks on the diet, 20 of 50 exposed mice developed mammary tumors as compared with 37 of 50 controls. (The subcommittee felt that the reduction in mammary neoplasms in the exposed mice was probably related to reduced body weight rather than to a true protective effect of fluoride.) The authors also evaluated the tumor-promoting effects of fluoride by administering sodium fluoride in the diets of mice after subcutaneous injection of 0.15 mg of benzopyrene. After 52 weeks, 13 of 40 fluoride-exposed mice developed sarcomas, as compared with 7 of 40 controls. In contrast, there was a marked reduction in the incidence of primary lung tumors in fluoride-exposed Swiss and ABC mice after 60-62 weeks of treatment. The authors were unable to provide a simple explanation for the divergent effects of sodium fluoride on subcutaneous sarcomas and lung tumors induced by benzopyrene.

Taylor (1954) exposed female DBA and C3H mice to low concentrations of sodium fluoride in drinking water (fluoride at 0.4-10 mg/L) for 7-17 months. Each treatment group comprised 12-42 mice, most groups comprising 20 animals. Many of the groups were maintained on a chow diet that contained fluoride up to 20 mg/kg; the remaining groups were fed a diet containing a negligible amount of fluoride. Mortality was greater in the fluoride-exposed groups, although the cause of the early deaths of animals given fluoridated water was not generally given. Mammary adenocarcinomas were observed in both exposed and control groups; in total, 59% of the deaths of exposed animals during the course of these studies were considered to be due to those tumors, as compared with 54% of the controls. The four groups of mice exposed to fluoride at 10 mg/L of drinking water averaged 63% mortality from cancer (all types of neoplasms combined) in comparison with 51% of the controls. The authors concluded that those data provided no indication that the incidence of cancer was increased as a result of exposure to fluoride. Despite the negative findings, the subcommittee felt that the study was inadequate because of the comparatively small number of animals assigned to each treatment group and the relatively short period of observation. The fluoride doses used in this study were also appreciably lower than current estimates of the maximum tolerated dose for fluoride (Bucher et al., 1991; Maurer et al., 1990, in press).

Taylor and Taylor (1965) showed that low concentrations of sodium fluoride can increase the rate of growth of transplanted mammary adenocarcinomas in DBA mice. In the study, sodium fluoride was added to the tumor tissue suspension before transplantation, to the drinking water of the host animals after transplantation, or by subdermal injection after transplantation. Acceleration of tumor growth was also demonstrated with tissue cultured in the yolk sacs of embryonated eggs. Tumor growth was enhanced by more than 100% in both cases. However, with exposure to higher concentrations of sodium fluoride, tumor growth was inhibited. The subcommittee observed that this model is unusual for studying tumor growth and noted the incongruous results at high and low levels of exposure.

Kanisawa and Schroeder (1969) exposed white Swiss mice of the Charles River strain (CD-1) to fluoride at 10 mg/L (administered as sodium fluoride) in drinking water for life. Male mice exposed to fluoride survived 1-2 months longer than unexposed controls. Ten percent of the males were still alive at 752 days of age; female mortality did not reach 90% until 789 days of age. Pathology examination was limited to a small number of tissues and macroscopically visible tumors. Of the 72 animals exposed to fluoride, 22 developed neoplasms (five of these were malignant) primarily in the lung. The lifetime incidence of specific tumors observed in those animals was comparable to that in the 71 controls. The authors concluded that oral ingestion of fluoride cannot be considered carcinogenic in mice at the dose given. The subcommittee felt that exposure was not adequately documented, particularly with respect to fluoride concentrations in bone. The pathological evaluation was also inadequate because bone lesions were not adequately assessed.

Recent Carcinogenicity Bioassays

Two recent studies have raised some concern about the ability of fluoride to induce cancer in animals. The study conducted by NTP (NTP, 1990; Bucher et al., 1991) indicated a possible increase in the incidence of osteosarcomas in F344/N male rats, although no such lesions were observed in female rats. B6C3F$_1$ mice also failed to demonstrate a carcinogenic response to fluoride.

The incidence of osteosarcomas in male and female rats in the study is shown in Table 7-2. Sodium fluoride was administered in the drinking water at concentrations of 25, 100, and 175 mg/L for 103 weeks. Fifty animals of each sex were assigned to the two lowest-dose groups, and 80 were assigned to the high-dose and control groups. Mild fluorosis was observed in teeth of all dose groups of both mice and rats, although more so in rats. Four osteosarcomas were observed in male rats: one in the group exposed to 100 mg/L and three in the group exposed to 175 mg/L. Two of the three osteosarcomas in the high-dose group were detected with radiographs. Although the incidence of osteosarcomas in the high-dose group was not significant ($p > 0.05$) in relation to the control

TABLE 7-2 Incidence of Oteosarcomas in Rats Exposed to Sodium Fluoride in Drinking Water

Rats	Concentration, mg/L	No. of Animals	No. of Osteosarcomas
Males	0	80	0
	25	51	0
	100	50	1
	175	80	3
Females	0	80	0
	25	50	0
	100	50	0
	175	81	0

Source: NTP, 1990.

response rate, the trend in response to increased dose was significant ($p = 0.027$). NTP considered those data "equivocal evidence of carcinogenic activity" in male rats, and "no evidence of carcinogenicity" in female rats or in male or female mice. The subcommittee felt that the study was generally well conducted in accordance with current bioassay standards and agreed with the interpretation of the results in isolation. However, the subcommittee also felt that the results must be examined in conjunction with results of other studies, particularly those of Maurer et al. (1990, in press).

The Maurer et al. (1990, in press) studies for Procter & Gamble (P&G) clearly indicated that sodium fluoride increased the incidence of osteomas (noncancerous bone tumors) in male and female CD-1 mice (Table 7-3) but not in male and female Sprague-Dawley rats. In the experiments, 60 female and 60 male mice and 70 female and 70 male rats were exposed to dietary sodium fluoride at concentrations of 4, 10, or 25 mg/kg of body weight per day. The length of the rat study, 95 weeks for males and 99 weeks for females, was based on a termination criterion of 20% survival. In the mice study, the 20% survival rate was reached at 95 weeks for males and 97 weeks for females.

Fluoride exposure induced severe fluorosis of bones and teeth in mice and rats and osteomas in both sexes of mice. The investigators cautioned that the increase in osteomas in mice might have resulted from a con-

2000

TABLE 7-3 Incidence of Osteomas in Male and Female CD-1 Mice Exposed
to Sodium Fluoride in Their Diet

Mice	Concentration, mg/kg	No. of Animals	No. of Animals with Osteomas[a]	No. of Osteosarcomas
Male	0	50	1	0
	0	45	0	0
	4	42	0	0
	10	44	2	0
	25	50	13	0
Females	0	50	2	0
	0	45	3	0
	4	42	4	0
	10	44	2	0
	25	50	13	0

[a]Historical control incidence in CD-1 mice is < 1%.
Source: Maurer et al., in press.

taminating retrovirus. The subcommittee noted, however, that the virus
would have to preferentially affect the exposed groups in relation to the
control groups to be solely responsible for the observed dose-response
relation. This point is discussed further below.

In attempting to resolve the apparent differences between the NTP and
P&G studies, several issues need to be considered.

• Different routes of exposure were used in the NTP and P&G studies. To evaluate the different results for rats in the two studies, a common measure of dose is needed. Doses in the two studies can be compared by using bone fluoride concentrations. Under the exposure conditions imposed in both studies (continuous exposure to fluoride in water
or feed), fluoride concentration in bone represents the most reliable
indicator of the total body burden of fluoride. Using that indicator, the
highest dose used in the P&G study was 2 to 3 times greater than the
highest dose used in the NTP study (Table 7-4) and yet it did not induce
bone neoplasms. Doses of fluoride at 4 mg/kg in feed in the P&G study
resulted in bone-ash fluoride concentrations comparable to those in the

TABLE 7-4 Comparison of NTP and P&G Studies

Fluoride Dose	Fluorde Concentrations in Bone Ash (μg of fluoride/mg of bone ash)			
	Rats		Mice	
	Males	Females	Males	Females
	NTP Study			
Control	445 (0)[a]	554 (0)	719 (0)	917 (0)
25 mg/L	978 (0)	1,348 (0)	1,606 (0)	1,523 (0)
100 mg/L	3,648 (1)	3,726 (0)	3,585 (0)	4,370 (0)
175 mg/L	5,263 (3)[b]	5,554 (0)	5,690 (0)	6,241 (0)
	P&G Study			
Control 1	467 (0)	505 (0)	1,582 (1)	971 (2)
Control 2	691 (0)	785 (0)	1,676 (0)	1,295 (3)
4 mg/kg	5,014 (0)	4,541 (0)	4,405 (0)	3,380 (4)
10 mg/kg	8,849 (0)	8,254 (0)	7,241 (2)	6,189 (2)
25 mg/kg	16,761 (0)	14,428 (0)	13,177 (13)[c]	10,572 (13)[c]

[a]Number in parenthesis is the number of osteosarcomas (in NTP study) or osteomas (in P&G study).
[b]Equivocal evidence of increased incidence of osteosarcomas (Bucher et al., 1991).
[c]Increased incidence of osteomas (Maurer et al., in press).

highest-dose group (NaF at 175 mg/L of drinking water) in the NTP study.

• It is important to evaluate the NTP finding of equivocal evidence of carcinogenic activity in male rats in the context of other studies. Such a weight-of-the-evidence approach is necessary to make an overall judgment concerning fluoride carcinogenicity. Even though the four earlier animal studies each suffered from deficiencies in design or interpretation, none gave any indication of an association between fluoride and osteosarcoma. Collectively, they provide limited support for the hypothesis of no association between exposure to fluoride and increased risk of osteosarcoma.

Even though the highest dose of fluoride in the P&G rat study was more than twice the highest dose in the NTP study in terms of bone fluoride concentrations (Table 7-4), no osteosarcomas were observed in either sex of rats in the P&G study. Therefore, the P&G study does not support the equivocal findings in the NTP study. However, different rat strains were used in these two studies; therefore, possible differences in susceptibility in these two strains cannot be ruled out.

• The role of the retrovirus in the P&G mouse studies is not clear. Because the virus is transmitted vertically, mice in all dose groups were infected. Also, there is no evidence that viral infection was linked to the occurrence of osteomas. An association between this retrovirus and osteoma has not been previously established: therefore, the subcommittee sees no convincing evidence that the retrovirus alone caused the osteomas. The virus might conceivably have had a potentiating effect on the induction of osteomas, although evidence for that is lacking. The subcommittee believes that the most obvious explanation for the increased incidence of osteomas in mice is that the dose in the P&G study (based on bone fluoride concentrations) was more than twice as high as the dose in the NTP study (Table 7-4) and that the occurrence of osteoma in the P&G study was related to exposure to fluoride.

• Of equal importance is the relevance of the mouse osteomas in terms of their relation to the potential carcinogenic activity of fluoride in animals and, by extension, in humans. The subcommittee considered the biological importance of the osteomas observed in mice in the P&G study from several perspectives. Are they part of a neoplastic continuum? Do they have the potential for malignant change? Should they be considered evidence of carcinogenic activity? Should they be considered a hyperplastic response? Are they a unique lesion induced by exposure to fluoride?

A critical issue in the P&G mouse study is whether the osteomas observed at the highest dose in male and female mice are related to osteosarcomas or to other neoplastic diseases. In an attempt to answer that and other questions, the subcommittee asked the Armed Forces Institute of Pathology (AFIP) to review the osteomas in the P&G study (Appendix 2). The results of their review are in Appendix 3.

According to the AFIP, arguments that support the view that the osteomas are not true neoplasms include the following: (1) none of the lesions progressed beyond the benign condition; (2) none of the tumors showed characteristics of precancerous change; (3) in contrast to primary bone neoplasms, which are usually unicentric in origin (in animals as well as humans), many of the osteomas in mice were multicentric; and (4) there is no human counterpart to this lesion.

• In the scientific community, there are clear differences in opinion concerning the relevance of high-dose toxicological studies in rodents to humans (Rall, 1991; Ames, 1991). Factors to be considered include the relative bone and plasma fluoride concentrations in animals exhibiting lesions in relation to the concentrations observed in human populations. Another factor to be considered is the relative plasma fluoride concentrations. Unfortunately, reliable plasma fluoride values are not available from the NTP study.

Suppose that, on the basis of the results of the NTP study, fluoride induces osteosarcoma in male rats at concentrations of approximately 5,300 ppm in bone ash. The bone-ash concentrations in mice where osteomas appeared to be related to fluoride exposure were approximately 13,200 ppm in males and 10,500 ppm in females (Table 7-4).

Studies of fluoride in human bone ash indicate that concentrations in people 70 years of age and older might exceed 4,000 ppm in exceptional cases where exposure to fluoride has been high. Osteosarcoma occurs in humans almost exclusively in the first three decades of life. Bone-ash concentrations in people of that age are substantially lower, generally less than 3,000 ppm.

Osteosarcoma is associated with long-bone growth in humans. The long bones cease to grow in teenaged humans but continue to grow throughout the lifetime of rats. Thus, rats are susceptible for a longer portion of their lifespan than humans. In fact, the osteosarcomas observed in the NTP study were found exclusively in older rats.

CONCLUSIONS

More than 50 epidemiological studies have been conducted to evaluate the relation between fluoride concentrations in drinking water and human cancer. With minor exceptions, these studies used the method of geographic or temporal comparisons of fluoridation status and regional cancer rates. There is no consistent observation of increased cancer risk with drinking-water fluoridation; most of the studies show no association. The large number of epidemiological studies combined with their lack of positive findings implies that if any link exists, it must be very weak.

Based on the weight of the available evidence, the subcommittee believes that the collective data from the rodent fluoride toxicological studies do not present convincing evidence of an association between fluoride and increased occurrence of bone cancer in animals. The equivocal result of osteosarcoma in male rats in the NTP study was not supported by results in females in the same study or by the P&G rat study, even though the latter had much higher exposure levels. That suggests that the male rat osteosarcomas observed in the NTP study were not related to fluoride exposure. The subcommittee concluded that the increased incidence of osteomas in male and female mice in the P&G study is most likely related to fluoride, although the presence of a contaminating retrovirus was considered a confounding factor. Consideration was given to the biological significance of the treatment-related increased incidence of benign osteomas in male and female mice at the highest dose in the P&G study. The key question is whether the osteomas are true neoplasms or not. The AFIP concluded that these lesions are not true bone neoplasms, and, therefore, it would be inappropriate to use them to establish carcinogenic activity. In fact, they are more reminiscent of hyperplastic (hyperostoses) than neoplastic lesions. The subcommittee concluded that the osteomas observed in mice at the highest dose in the P&G study are of questionable biological significance in terms of their relevance to humans, especially in light of their occurrence at fluoride exposures far greater than those that are likely to occur in humans.

The subcommittee concludes that the available laboratory data are insufficient to demonstrate a carcinogenic effect of fluoride in animals. The subcommittee also concludes that the weight of the evidence from more than 50 epidemiological studies does not support the hypothesis of an association between fluoride exposure and increased cancer risk in humans.

RECOMMENDATIONS

The subcommittee observed that weak associations between cancer risk and exposure to fluoride, if they exist, might be more readily identified in analytical studies based on individual outcome and exposure information than in ecological studies based on aggregate outcomes and exposures. Thus, conducting well-designed studies with information from individuals is important in the ongoing evaluation of fluoride carcinogenicity. The subcommittee therefore recommends conducting one or more highly focused, carefully designed analytical studies (case control or cohort) of the cancer sites that are most highly suspect, based on data from animal studies and the few suggestions of a carcinogenic effect reported in the epidemiological literature. Such studies should be designed to gather information on individual study subjects so that adjustments can be made for the potential confounding effects of other risk factors in analyses of individuals. Information on fluoride exposure from sources other than water must be obtained, and estimates of exposure from drinking water should be as accurate as possible. In addition, analysis of fluoride in bone samples from patients and controls would be valuable in inferring total lifetime exposure to fluoride. Among the disease outcomes that warrant separate study are osteosarcomas and cancers of the buccal cavity, kidney, and bones and joints.

8 INTAKE, METABOLISM, AND DISPOSITION OF FLUORIDE

FLUORIDE INTAKE

The literature contains several reviews of the sources and amounts of fluoride intake by age, water fluoride concentration, and geographic region in the United States that may be consulted for detailed discussions (McClure, 1943; Farkas and Farkas, 1974; Myers, 1978; Ophaug et al., 1980a,b, 1985; Whitford, 1989; Burt, 1992). This discussion will summarize our current understanding of the main points covered in those reports.

The major sources of fluoride intake are water, beverages, food, and fluoride-containing dental products. Fluoride exposure from the atmosphere generally accounts for a small fraction (about 0.01 mg per day) of the intake of fluoride (Hodge and Smith, 1977). The fluoride concentrations in groundwater range from less than 0.1 mg/L to more than 100 mg/L and depend mainly on the concentration and solubility of fluoride compounds in the soil. The fluoride concentrations in foods also depend on the fluoride concentrations in soil but can be increased or decreased according to the fluoride concentrations in water used for preparation. The fluoride concentrations in most dental products available in the United States range from 230 ppm (0.05% sodium fluoride mouth rinse) to over 12,000 ppm (1.23% acidulated phosphate fluoride gel).

125

The average intake of dietary fluoride by young children who drink water containing fluoride at 0.7-1.2 mg/L is approximately 0.5 mg per day or 0.04-0.07 mg/kg of body weight per day, although substantial variation occurs among individuals (McClure, 1943; Ophaug et al., 1980a,b, 1985). The classical epidemiological studies done in the 1930s and 1940s on the relation between water fluoride concentrations and dental caries and dental fluorosis determined that 0.7-1.2 mg/L was optimal because it provided a high degree of protection against dental caries and a low prevalence of milder forms of dental fluorosis. Thus, the associated amount of intake by children (0.04-0.07 mg/kg per day) has generally been accepted as optimal, or as Burt (1992) has said, as "a useful upper limit for fluoride intake by children."

Fluoride intake by nursing infants depends mainly on whether breast milk or formula is fed. Human breast milk contains only a trace of fluoride (about 0.5 μmol/L, depending on fluoride intake) and provides less than 0.01 mg of fluoride per day (Ekstrand et al., 1984). Ready-to-feed formulas generally contain fluoride at less than 0.4 mg/L (Johnson and Bawden, 1987; McKnight-Hanes et al., 1988), and formulas reconstituted with fluoridated water (0.7-1.2 mg/L) contain fluoride at 0.7 mg/L or more. Thus, fluoride intake from formula might range from less than 0.4 to over 1.0 mg per day. It is evident that that range includes amounts that exceed the optimal range of 0.7-1.2 mg/L and, therefore, might be thought to increase the risk of dental fluorosis. Recent evidence, however, indicates that the transitional or early-maturation stage of enamel development is when the tissue is most susceptible to fluoride-induced changes (Evans, 1989; Pendrys and Stamm, 1990; Evans and Stamm, 1991a). The early-maturation stage occurs during the third or fourth year of life for the permanent anterior teeth when the amount of dietary fluoride intake in a community with fluoridated water is generally within 0.04-0.07 mg/kg per day.

Ophaug et al. (1980a,b) determined dietary fluoride intake by young children in four regions of the United States. Mean intake by 6-month-old infants was 0.21-0.54 mg per day, and that by 2-year-old children was 0.32-0.61 mg per day. The mean intake by the 2-year-old children (but not the 6-month-old group) was directly related to the fluoride concentration in the drinking water. Those data are in close agreement with the findings of Dabeka et al. (1982) and Featherstone and Shields (1988). Dietary fluoride intake by adults living in areas served with water fluoridated at about 1.0 mg/L has been estimated at 1.2 mg per day

(Singer et al., 1980), 1.8 mg per day (Taves, 1983), and 2.2 mg per day (San Filippo and Battistone, 1971). Intake by some people, such as outdoor laborers in warm climates or those with high urine output disorders (Klein, 1975), would be substantially higher. Fluoride-containing dental products intended for topical application of fluoride to teeth (especially toothpastes because of their widespread use) are an important source of ingested fluoride for both children and adults. Dowell (1981) reported that nearly 50% of his sample had started brushing by the age of 12 months. At 18 months, 75% were brushing with fluoride toothpaste. The average amount of toothpaste used in one brushing is 1.0 g (ranging from 0.1 to 2.0 g), which, for a product at 1,000 ppm, contains 1.0 mg of fluoride. The results from several studies indicate that an average of 25% (ranging from 10% to 100%) of fluoride introduced into the mouth with toothpaste or mouth rinse is ingested, but the percentage is higher for young children who do not have good control of the swallowing reflex (Hellström, 1960; Ericsson and Forsman, 1969; Hargreaves et al., 1972; Parkins, 1972; Barnhart et al., 1974; Baxter, 1980; Dowell, 1981; Wei and Kanellis, 1983; Bell et al., 1985; Bruun and Thylstrup, 1988). It has been calculated that the amount of fluoride ingested with toothpaste (or mouth rinse) by children who live in a community with optimally fluoridated water, who have good control of swallowing, and who brush (or rinse) twice a day is approximately equal to the daily intake of fluoride with food, water, and beverages (Whitford et al., 1987). In the case of younger children or those who, for any other reason, have poor control of swallowing, the daily intake of fluoride from dental products could exceed dietary intake.

For several reasons, differences in fluoride intake in communities with different water fluoride concentrations are likely to be smaller today than in the 1940s, when the epidemiological studies of dental caries and fluorosis studies by H.T. Dean and his associates were done. The use of fluoride-containing dental products, especially toothpastes, is widespread, and dietary fluoride supplements are prescribed for children from birth to teenage years more frequently in areas without water fluoridation. The dosage schedule for fluoride supplementation currently recommended by the American Dental Association and the American Academy of Pediatrics is shown in Table 8-1. Furthermore, most urban areas in many states have controlled water fluoride concentrations (about 1.0 mg/L). In general, the so-called "halo effect" occurs in those areas where foods and beverages are processed and packaged for distribution

TABLE 8-1 Dietary Fluoride Supplementation Schedule Recommended by the American Dental Association and the American Academy of Pediatrics

Age Group, yr	Drinking-Water Fluoride Concentration, mg/L		
	<0.3	0.3-0.7	>0.7
Recommended amount[a] from birth to 2	0.25	0	0
Recommended amount from 2 to 3	0.50	0.25	0
Recommended amount from 3 to 13	1.0	0.50	0

[a]Values are given in milligrams of fluoride per day (2.2 mg of NaF and 1.0 mg of fluoride).

to other communities, including those without fluoridated water supplies. At the expense of tap-water consumption, soft-drink consumption in the United States and Canada has increased sharply in recent years in both fluoridated and nonfluoridated areas (Beals et al., 1981; Chao et al., 1984; Ismail et al., 1984; Clovis and Hargreaves, 1988). Fluoride intake from soft drinks and other beverages prepared with fluoridated water amounts to 0.3-0.5 mg per 12 ounces, which makes such products quantitatively important sources of fluoride.

Those considerations and others, such as use of certain home-water purification systems that might remove fluoride and consumption of bottled water that might have fluoride concentrations above or below the optimal range, lead to the conclusion that reasonably accurate estimates of total daily fluoride intake are no longer as simple and straightforward as they were when the only important source of fluoride was water. Investigators seeking to examine the possible relation between fluoride intake and health outcomes, such as dental caries, fluorosis, or quality of bone, need to be aware of the complex situation that exists today. It is no longer feasible to estimate with reasonable accuracy the level of fluoride exposure simply on the basis of concentration in drinking water supply.

FLUORIDE ABSORPTION

Approximately 75-90% of the fluoride ingested each day is absorbed from the alimentary tract. The half-time for absorption is approximately

30 minutes, so peak plasma concentrations usually occur within 30-60 minutes. Absorption across the oral mucosa is limited and probably accounts for less than 1% of the daily intake. Absorption from the stomach occurs readily and is inversely related to the pH of the gastric contents (Whitford and Pashley, 1984). Most of the fluoride that enters the intestine will be absorbed rapidly. It was generally believed that fluoride excreted in the feces was never absorbed, although several studies with rats (G.M. Whitford, Medical College of Georgia, Augusta, unpublished data, 1992) indicate that a diet high in calcium or parenteral administration of fluoride can result in fecal fluoride excretion rates that exceed fluoride intake. High concentrations of dietary calcium and other cations that form insoluble complexes with fluoride can reduce fluoride absorption from the gastrointestinal tract.

The mechanism of fluoride absorption has received considerable research attention and has led to the conclusion that diffusion is the underlying process. Absorption across the oral and gastric mucosae is strongly pH-dependent. That finding is consistent with the hypothesis that hydrofluoric acid ($pK_a = 3.4$) is the permeating moiety. Results from studies with rats indicate that fluoride absorption across the intestinal mucosa is not pH-dependent (Nopakun and Messer, 1989).

FLUORIDE IN PLASMA

There are two general forms of fluoride in human plasma. The ionic form is the one of interest in dentistry, medicine, and public health. Ionic fluoride is detectable by the ion-specific electrode. It is not bound to proteins or other components of plasma or to soft tissues. The other form consists of several fat-soluble organic fluorocompounds. These can be contaminants derived from food processing and packaging. Perfluoro-octanoic acid (octanoic acid fully substituted with fluoride) has been identified as one of the fluorocompounds (Guy, 1979). The biological fate and importance of the organic fluorocompounds remains largely unknown. The extent to which the fluorine in these compounds is exchangeable with the ionic fluoride pool has not been determined. The concentration of ionic fluoride in soft and hard tissues is directly related to the amount of ionic fluoride intake, but that of the fluorocompounds is not. Neither form is homeostatically controlled (Guy, 1979; Whitford and Williams, 1986).

Provided that water is the major source of fluoride intake, fasting plasma fluoride concentrations of healthy young or middle-aged adults expressed as micromoles per liter are roughly equal to the fluoride concentrations in drinking water expressed as milligrams per liter. Plasma fluoride concentrations, however, tend to increase slowly over the years until the sixth or seventh decade of life when they, like fluoride concentrations in bone, tend to increase more rapidly. The reason for that change is uncertain but might be due to declining renal function or increasing resorption of bone crystals with low fluoride concentrations (leaving an increased density of crystals with high fluoride concentrations). Cord-blood plasma concentrations are 75-80% as high as maternal plasma concentrations, indicating that fluoride freely crosses the placenta (Shen and Taves, 1974). The balance of fluoride in the neonate can be positive or negative during the early months of life, depending on whether intake is sufficient to maintain the plasma concentration that existed at the time of birth (Ekstrand et al., 1984).

TISSUE DISTRIBUTION

As indicated by the results of short-term ^{18}F isotope studies with rats, a steady-state distribution exists between the fluoride concentrations in plasma or extracellular fluid and the intracellular fluid of most soft tissues (Whitford et al., 1979). Intracellular fluoride concentrations are lower, but they change proportionately and simultaneously with those of plasma. With the exception of the kidney, which concentrates fluoride within the renal tubules, tissue-to-plasma (T/P) fluoride ratios are less than 1.0. In those cases in which the T/P ratio exceeds unity, as might occur in the aorta or the placenta near term, ectopic calcification should be suspected. Most of the published data on soft-tissue concentrations in humans were obtained with analytical methods that were insensitive and nonspecific or that had excessively high blanks. Further work is needed using modern analytical techniques, such as the ion-specific electrode after isolation of fluoride with the hexamethyldisiloxane-facilitated diffusion method of Taves (1968) and modified by Whitford (1989). Venkateswarlu (1990) described and compared the merits of a variety of analytical methods for the determination of fluoride.

The fluoride concentrations of several of the specialized body fluids, including gingival crevicular fluid, ductal saliva, bile, and urine, are also related to those of plasma in a steady-state manner. The fluoride concentrations of breast milk and cerebrospinal fluid tend to be related to those of plasma, but they respond slowly to changes in plasma fluoride concentrations (Spak et al., 1983).

The mechanism underlying the transmembrane migration of fluoride appears to be the diffusion equilibrium of hydrogen fluoride (Whitford, 1989). Thus, factors that change the magnitude of transmembrane or transepithelial pH gradients will affect the tissue distribution of fluoride accordingly. In general, epithelia and cell membranes of most tissues appear to be essentially impermeable to the fluoride ion, which is charged and has a large hydrated radius.

Approximately 99% of the body burden of fluoride is associated with calcified tissues. Of the fluoride absorbed by the young or middle-aged adult each day, approximately 50% will be associated with calcified tissues within 24 hours and the remainder will be excreted in urine. This 50:50 distribution is shifted strongly in favor of greater retention in the very young. Increased retention is due to the large surface area provided by numerous and loosely organized developing bone crystallites, which increase the clearance rate of fluoride from plasma by the skeleton (Whitford, 1989). Accordingly, the peak plasma fluoride concentrations and the areas under the time-plasma concentration curves are directly related to age during the period of skeletal development. Due to decreased accretion and increased resorption of bone, the 50:50 distribution is probably shifted in favor of greater excretion in the later years of life, but less is known about that.

Fluoride is strongly but not irreversibly bound to apatite and other calcium phosphate compounds that might be present in calcified tissues. In the short term, fluoride might be mobilized from the hydration shells and the surfaces of bone crystallites (and presumably dentin and developing enamel crystallites) by isoionic or heteroionic exchange. In the long term, the ion is mobilized by the normal process of bone remodeling. Waterhouse et al. (1980) reported that human serum fluoride concentrations were increased following administration of Parathormone and decreased by administration of calcitonin.

FLUORIDE EXCRETION

Elimination of absorbed fluoride from the body occurs almost exclusively via the kidneys. As noted above, about 10-25% of the daily intake of fluoride is not absorbed and remains to be excreted in feces. Data from the 1940s indicated that the amount of fluoride excreted in sweat could nearly equal urinary fluoride excretion under hot moist conditions (McClure et al., 1945). More recent data obtained with modern analytical techniques (G.M. Whitford, Medical College of Georgia, Augusta, unpublished data, 1992), however, indicate that sweat fluoride concentrations are very low and similar to those of plasma (about 1-3 μmol/L). Therefore, sweat is probably a quantitatively minor route for fluoride excretion under even extreme environmental conditions.

The clearance rate of fluoride from plasma is essentially equal to the sum of the clearances by calcified tissues and kidneys. The renal clearances of chloride, iodide, and bromide in healthy young or middle-aged adults are typically less than 1.0 mL per minute, but the renal clearance of fluoride is approximately 35 mL per minute (Waterhouse et al., 1980; Cowell and Taylor, 1981; Schiffl and Binswanger, 1982). Little is known about the renal handling of fluoride by infants, young children, and the elderly. A 600-day longitudinal study of fluoride pharmacokinetics that began with weanling dogs, however, indicated that the renal clearance of fluoride factored by body weight (milliliter per minute per kilogram) was independent of age (Whitford, 1989). In patients with compromised renal function where the glomerular filtration rate falls to 30% of normal on a chronic basis, fluoride excretion might decline sufficiently to result in increased soft- and hard-tissue fluoride concentrations (Schiffl and Binswanger, 1980). Renal handling, tissue concentrations, and effects of fluoride in renal patients are subjects in need of further research.

Fluoride is freely filtered through the glomerular capillaries and undergoes tubular reabsorption in varying degrees. There is no evidence for net tubular secretion or a tubular transport maximum of the ion. The renal clearance of fluoride is directly related to urinary pH (Whitford et al., 1976) and, under some conditions, to urinary flow rate (Chen et al., 1956). Recent data from stop-flow studies with dogs indicate that fluoride reabsorption is greatest from the distal nephron, the site where the tubular fluid is acidified (Whitford and Pashley, 1991). As in the cases of gastric absorption and transmembrane migration, the mechanism for the tubular reabsorption of fluoride appears to be the diffusion of hydrogen fluoride. Thus, factors that affect urinary pH such as diet, drugs, metabolic or respiratory disorders, and altitude of residence, have been shown or can be expected to affect the extent to which absorbed fluoride is retained in the body (Whitford, 1989).

RECOMMENDATIONS

Further research is needed in the following areas:

• Determine and compare the intake of fluoride from all sources, including fluoride-containing dental products, in fluoridated and non-fluoridated communities. That information would improve our understanding of trends in dental caries, dental fluorosis, and possibly other disorders or diseases.

• Determine the effects of factors that affect human acid-base balance and urinary pH on the metabolic characteristics, balance, and tissue concentrations of fluoride.

• Determine the metabolic characteristics of fluoride in infants, young children, and the elderly.

• Determine prospectively the metabolic characteristics of fluoride in patients with progressive renal disease.

• Using preparative and analytical methods now available, determine soft-tissue fluoride concentrations and their relation to plasma fluoride concentrations. Consider the relation of tissue concentrations to variables of interest, including past fluoride exposure and age.

• Identify the compounds that compose the "organic fluoride pool" in human plasma and determine their sources, metabolic characteristics, fate, and biological importance.

REFERENCES

Aardema, M.J., D.P. Gibson, and R.A. LeBoeuf. 1989. Sodium fluoride-induced chromosome aberrations in different stages of the cell cycle: A proposed mechanism. Mutat. Res. 223:191-203.

Aasenden, R. 1974. Fluoride concentrations in the surface tooth enamel of young men and women. Arch. Oral Biol. 19:697-701.

Adair, S.M. 1989. Risks and benefits of fluoride mouthrinsing. Pediatrician 16:161-169.

Al-Alousi, W., D. Jackson, G. Crompton, and O.C. Jenkins. 1975. Enamel mottling in a fluoride and in a non-fluoride community. Br. Dent. J. 138:9-15, 56-60.

Albanese, R. 1987. Sodium fluoride and chromosome damage (in vitro human lymphocyte and in vivo micronucleus assays). Mutagenesis 2:497-499.

Alm, P.E. 1983. Sodium fluoride-evoked histamine release from mast cells: A study of cyclic AMP levels and effects of catecholamines. Agents Actions 13:132-137.

Ames, B.N. 1991. Response to 'Carcinogens and human health: Part 2' [letter]. Science 251:12-13.

Angmar-Månsson, B., and G.M. Whitford. 1982. Plasma fluoride levels and enamel fluorosis in the rat. Caries Res. 16:334-339.

Angmar-Månsson, B., and G.M. Whitford. 1984. Enamel fluorosis related to plasma F levels in the rat. Caries Res. 18:25-32.

Angmar-Månsson, B., and G.M. Whitford. 1985. Single fluoride doses and enamel fluorosis in the rat. Caries Res. 19:145-152.

Angmar-Månsson, B., and G.M. Whitford. 1990. Environmental and physiological factors affecting dental fluorosis. J. Dent. Res. 69(Spec. Issue):706-713.

Angmar-Månsson, B., Y. Ericsson, and O. Ekberg. 1976. Plasma fluoride and enamel fluorosis. Calcif. Tiss. Res. 22:77-84.

Angmar-Månsson, B., U. Lindh, and G.M. Whitford. 1990. Enamel and dentin fluoride levels and fluorosis following single fluoride doses: A nuclear microprobe study. Caries Res. 24:258-262.

Araibi, A.A.A., W.H. Yousif, and O.S. Al-Dewachi. 1989. Effect of high fluoride on the reproductive performance of the male rat. J. Biol. Sci. Res. 20:19-30.

Arends, J., and J. Christoffersen. 1990. Nature and role of loosely bound fluoride in dental caries. J. Dent. Res. 69(Spec. Issue):601-605.

Arlauskas, A., R.S.U. Baker, A.M. Bonin, R.K. Tandon, P.T. Crisp, and J. Ellis. 1985. Mutagenicity of metal ions in bacteria. Environ. Res. 36:379-388.

Arnold, F.A., Jr., H.T. Dean, and J.W. Knutson. 1953. Effect of fluoridated public water supplies on dental caries prevalence. Public Health Rep. 68:141-148.

Arnold, F.A., Jr., F.J. McClure, and C.L. White. 1960. Sodium fluoride tablets for children. Dental Prog. 1:8-12.

Ast, D.B., and H.C. Chase. 1953. The Newburgh-Kingston caries fluorine study. IV. Dental findings after six years of fluoridation. Oral Surg. Oral Med. Oral Pathol. 6:114-123.

Ast, D.B., D.J. Smith, B. Wachs, and K.T. Cantwell. 1956. Newburgh-Kingston caries-fluorine study. XIV. Combined clinical and roentgenographic dental findings after ten years of fluoride experience. J. Am. Dent. Assoc. 52:314-325.

Aulerich, R.J., A.C. Napolitano, S.J. Bursian, B.A. Olson, and J.R. Hochstein. 1987. Chronic toxicity of dietary fluorine to mink. J. Anim. Sci. 65:1759-1767.

Austen, K.F., M. Dworetzky, R.S. Farr, G.B. Logan, S. Malkiel, E. Middleton, Jr., M.M. Miller, R. Patterson, C.E. Reed, S.C. Siegel, P.P. van Arsdel, Jr. 1971. A statement on the question of allergy to fluoride used in the fluoridation of community water supplies. J. Allergy 47:347-348.

Backer Dirks, O. 1967. The relation between the fluoridation of water and dental caries experience. Int. Dent. J. 17:582-605.

Backer Dirks, O., B. Houwink, and G.W. Kwant. 1961. The results of 6 1/2 years of artificial fluoridation of drinking water in The Netherlands: The Tiel-Culemborg experiment. Arch. Oral Biol. 5:284-300.

Bælum, V., O. Fejerskov, F. Manji, and M.J. Larsen. 1987. Daily dose of fluoride and dental fluorosis. Tandlægebladet 91:452-456.

Bagramian, R.A., S. Narendran, and M. Ward. 1989. Relationship of dental caries and fluorosis to fluoride supplement history in a non-fluoridated sample of schoolchildren. Adv. Dent. Res. 3:161-167.

Bale, S.S., and M.T. Mathew. 1987. Analysis of chromosomal abnormalities at anaphase-telophase induced by sodium fluoride in vitro. Cytologia 52:889-893.

Barnhart, W.E., L.K. Hiller, G.J. Leonard, and S.E. Michaels. 1974. Dentifrice usage and ingestion among four age groups. J. Dent. Res. 53:1317-1322.

Baxter, P.M. 1980. Toothpaste ingestion during toothbrushing by school children. Br. Dent. J. 148:125-128.

Beals, T.L., G.H. Anderson, R.D. Peterson, G.W. Thompson, and J.A. Hargreaves. 1981. Between-meal eating by Ontario children and teenagers. J. Can. Diet. Assoc. 42:242-247.

Beary, D.F. 1969. The effects of fluoride and low calcium on the physical properties of the rat femur. Anat. Rec. 164:305-316.

Bell, R.A., G.M. Whitford, J.T. Barenie, and D.R. Myers. 1985. Fluoride retention in children using self-applied topical fluoride products. Clin. Prev. Dent. 7(3):22-27.

Beltran, E.D., and B.A. Burt. 1988. The pre- and posteruptive effects of fluoride in the caries decline. J. Public Health Dent. 48:233-240.

Black, G.V., and F.S. McKay. 1916. Mottled teeth: An endemic developmental imperfection of the enamel of the teeth heretofore unknown in the literature of dentistry. Dent. Cosmos 58:129-156.

Bohaty, B.S., W.A. Parker, N.S. Seale, and E.R. Zimmerman. 1989. The prevalence of fluorosis-like lesions associated with topical and systemic fluoride usage in an area of optimal water fluoridation. Pediatr. Dent. 11:125-128.

Bowden, G.H.W. 1990. Effects of fluoride on the microbial ecology of dental plaque. J. Dent. Res. 69(Spec. Issue):653–659.

Brunelle, J.A. 1989. The prevalence of dental fluorosis in U.S. children, 1987 [abstract]. J. Dent. Res. 68(Spec. Issue):995.

Brunelle, J.A., and J.P. Carlos. 1990. Recent trends in dental caries in U.S. children and the effect of water fluoridation. J. Dent. Res. 69(Spec. Issue):723–727.

Bruun, C., and A. Thylstrup. 1988. Dentifrice usage among Danish children. J. Dent. Res. 67:1114–1117.

Bucher, J.R., M.R. Hejtmancik, J.D. Toft II, R.L. Persing, S.L. Eustis, and J.K. Haseman. 1991. Results and conclusions of the National Toxicology Program's rodent carcinogenicity studies with sodium fluoride. Int. J. Cancer 48:733–737.

Büchi, R., and K. Bürki. 1975. The origin of chromosome aberrations in mature sperm of *Drosophila*: Influence of sodium fluoride on treatments with trenimon and 1-phenyl-3,3-dimethyltriazene. Arch. Genet. 48:59–67.

Burt, B.A. 1992. The changing patterns of systemic fluoride intake. J. Dent. Res. 71(Spec. Issue):1228–1237.

Butler, W., V. Segreto, and E. Collins. 1985a. Describing the severity of mottling in a community: A different approach. Community Dent. Oral Epidemiol. 13:277–280.

Butler, W.J., V. Segreto, and E. Collins. 1985b. Prevalence of dental mottling in school-aged lifetime residents of 16 Texas communities. Am. J. Public Health 75:1408–1412.

Carriere, D., E.M. Bird, and J.W. Stamm. 1987. Influence of a diet of fluoride-fed cockerels on reproductive performance of captive American kestrels. Environ. Pollut. 46:151–159.

Caspary, W.J., B. Myhr, L. Bowers, D. McGregor, C. Riach, and A. Brown. 1987. Mutagenic activity of fluorides in mouse lymphoma cells. Mutat. Res. 187:165–180.

Caspary, W.J., R. Langenbach, B.W. Penman, C. Crespi, B.C. Myhr, and A.D. Mitchell. 1988. The mutagenic activity of selected compounds at the TK locus: Rodent vs. human cells. Mutat. Res. 196: 61–81.

Cauley, J.A., P.A. Murphy, T. Riley, and D. Black. 1991. Public health bonus of water fluoridation: Does fluoridation prevent osteoporosis and its related fractures [abstract]? Am. J. Epidemiol. 134: 768.

Chandra, S., R. Sharma, V.P. Thergaonkar, and S.K. Chaturvedi. 1980. Determination of optimal fluoride concentration in drinking water in an area in India with dental fluorosis. Community Dent. Oral Epidemiol. 8:92-96.

Chao, E.S.M., G.H. Anderson, G.W. Thompson, J.A. Hargreaves, and R.D. Peterson. 1984. A longitudinal study of dietary changes of a sample of Ontario children. II. Food intake. J. Can. Diet. Assoc. 45:112-118.

Chen, P.S., Jr., F.A. Smith, D.E. Gardner, J.A. O'Brien, and H.C. Hodge. 1956. Renal clearance of fluoride. Proc. Soc. Exp. Biol. Med. 92:879-883.

Chibole, O. 1987. Epidemiology of dental fluorosis in Kenya. J. R. Soc. Health 107:242-243.

Chow, L.C. 1990. Tooth-bound fluoride and dental caries. J. Dent. Res. 69(Spec. Issue):595-600.

Clarkson, J. 1989. Review of terminology, classifications, and indices of developmental defects of enamel. Adv. Dent. Res. 3:104-109.

Clarkson, J., and D. O'Mullane. 1989. A modified DDE index for use in epidemiological studies of enamel defects. J. Dent. Res. 68: 445-450.

Cleaton-Jones, P., and J.A. Hargreaves. 1990. Comparison of three fluorosis indices in a Namibian community with twice optimum fluoride in the drinking water. J. Dent. Assoc. S. Afr. 45:173-175.

Clovis, J., and J.A. Hargreaves. 1988. Fluoride intake from beverage consumption. Community Dent. Oral Epidemiol. 16:11-15.

Cohn, P.D. 1992. A Brief Report on the Association of Drinking Water Fluoridation and the Incidence of Osteosarcoma Among Young Males. A report prepared for the New Jersey Department of Environmental Protection and Energy and the New Jersey Department of Health, Trenton, N.J.

Cole, J., W.J. Muriel, and B.A. Bridges. 1986. The mutagenicity of sodium fluoride to L5178Y [wild-type and $TK^{+/-}$ (3.7.2c)] mouse lymphoma cells. Mutagenesis 1:157-167.

Cooper, C., C.A.C. Wickham, D.J.R. Barker, and S.J. Jacobsen. 1991. Water fluoridation and hip fracture [letter]. JAMA 266:513-514.

Cowell, D.C., and W.H. Taylor. 1981. Ionic fluoride: A study of its physiological variation in man. Ann. Clin. Biochem. 18(Pt. 2):76-83.

Crespi, C.L., G.M. Seixas, T. Turner, and B.W. Penman. 1990. Sodium fluoride is a less efficient human cell mutagen at low concentrations. Environ. Mol. Mutagen. 15:71-77.

Cutress, T.W., and G.W. Suckling. 1990. Differential diagnosis of dental fluorosis. J. Dent. Res. 69(Spec. Issue):714-720.

Dabeka, R.W., A.D. McKenzie, H.B. Conacher, and D.C. Kirkpatrick. 1982. Determination of fluoride in Canadian infant foods and calculation of fluoride intakes by infants. Can. J. Public Health 73:188-191.

Dambacher, M.A., J. Ittner, and P. Ruegsegger. 1986. Long-term fluoride therapy of postmenopausal osteoporosis. Bone 7:199-205.

Danielson, C., J.L. Lyon, M. Egger, and G.K. Goodenough. 1992. Hip fractures and fluoridation in Utah's elderly population. JAMA 268:746-748.

Daston, G.P., B.F. Rehnberg, B. Carver, and R.J. Kavlock. 1985. Toxicity of sodium fluoride to the postnatally developing rat kidney. Environ. Res. 37:461-474.

Dawes, C. 1989. Fluorides: Mechanisms of action and recommendations for use. J. Can. Dent. Assoc. 55:721-723.

Dean, H.T. 1934. Classification of mottled enamel diagnosis. J. Am. Dent. Assoc. 21:1421-1426.

Dean, H.T. 1942. The investigation of physiological effects by the epidemiological method. Pp. 23-31 in Fluorine and Dental Health, AAAS Publ. No. 19, F.R. Moulton, ed. Washington, D.C.: American Association for the Advancement of Science.

Dean, H.T., P. Jay, F.A. Arnold, Jr., and E. Elvove. 1941. Domestic water and dental caries. II. A study of 2,832 white children aged 12-14 years, of 8 suburban Chicago communities, including *Lactobacillus acidophilus* studies of 1,761 children. Public Health Rep. 56:761-792.

Den Besten, P.K. 1986. Effects of fluoride on protein secretion and removal during enamel development in the rat. J. Dent. Res. 65: 1272-1277.

Den Besten, P.K., and M.A. Crenshaw. 1987. Studies on the changes in developing enamel caused by ingestion of high levels of fluoride in the rat. Adv. Dent. Res. 1:176-180.

Desai, V.K., B.S. Bhavsar, N.R. Mehta, D.K. Saxena, and S.L. Kantharia. 1986. Symptomatology of workers in the fluoride industry and fluorspar processing plants. Stud. Environ. Sci. 27:193-200.

Dooland, M.B., and A. Wylie. 1989. A photographic study of enamel defects among South Australian school children. Aust. Dent. J. 34:470-473.

Dowell, T.B. 1981. The use of toothpaste in infancy. Br. Dent. J. 150:247-249.

Driscoll, W.S., H.S. Horowitz, R.J. Meyers, S.B. Heifetz, A. Kingman, and E.R. Zimmerman. 1986. Prevalence of dental caries and dental fluorosis in areas with negligible, optimal, and above-optimal fluoride concentrations in drinking water. J. Am. Dent. Assoc. 113:29-33.

Dummer, P.M.H., A. Kingdon, and R. Kingdon. 1990. Prevalence and distribution by tooth type and surface of developmental defects of dental enamel in a group of 15- to 16-year-old children in South Wales. Community Dent. Health 7:369-377.

Dunipace, A.J., W. Zhang, T.W. Noblitt, Y. Li, and G.K. Stookey. 1989. Genotoxic evaluation of chronic fluoride exposure: Micronucleus and sperm morphology studies. J. Dent. Res. 68:1525-1528.

Easmann, R.P., D.E. Steflik, D.H. Pashley, R.V. McKinney, Jr., and G.M. Whitford. 1984. Surface changes in rat gastric mucosa induced by sodium fluoride: A scanning electron microscopic study. J. Oral Pathol. 13:255-264.

Easmann, R.P., D.H. Pashley, N.L. Birdsong, R.V. McKinney, Jr., and G.M. Whitford. 1985. Recovery of rat gastric mucosa following single fluoride dosing. J. Oral Pathol. 14:779-792.

Eckerlin, R.H., G.A. Maylin, and L. Krook. 1986a. Milk production of cows fed fluoride contaminated commerical feed. Cornell Vet. 76:403-414.

Eckerlin, R.H., L. Krook, G.A. Maylin, and D. Carmichael. 1986b. Toxic effects of food-borne fluoride in silver foxes. Cornell Vet. 76:395-402.

Eckerlin, R.H., G.A. Maylin, L. Krook, and D.T. Carmichael. 1988. Ameliorative effects of reduced food-borne fluoride on reproduction in silver foxes. Cornell Vet. 78:385-391.

Edwards, M.J., and J.M. Parry. 1986. Sodium fluoride mediated DNA damage and DNA replication in mammalian cells. Mutagenesis 1:77-78.

Einhorn, T.A., G.K. Wakley, S. Linkhart, E.B. Rush, S. Maloney, E. Faierman, and D.J. Baylink. 1992. Incorporation of sodium fluoride into cortical bone does not impair the mechanical properties of the appendicular skeleton in rats. Calcif. Tissue Int. 51:127-131.

Eklund, S.A., B.A. Burt, A.I. Ismail, and J.J. Calderone. 1987. High-fluoride drinking water, fluorosis, and dental caries in adults. J. Am. Dent. Assoc. 114:324-328.

Ekstrand, J., C.J. Spak, and M. Ehrnebo. 1982. Renal clearance of fluoride in a steady state condition in man: Influence of urinary flow and pH changes by diet. Acta Pharmacol. Toxicol. 50:321-325.

Ekstrand, J., L.I. Hardell, and C.J. Spak. 1984. Fluoride balance studies on infants in a 1-ppm-water-fluoride area. Caries Res. 18:87-92.

Englander, H.R., and P.F. DePaola. 1979. Enhanced anticaries action from drinking water containing 5 ppm fluoride. J. Am. Dent. Assoc. 98:35-39.

Ericsson, S.Y. 1977. Cariostatic mechanisms of fluorides: Clinical observations. Caries Res. 11(Suppl 1):2-41.

Ericsson, Y. and B. Forsman. 1969. Fluoride retained from mouth-rinses and dentifrices in preschool children. Caries Res. 3:290-299.

Evans, R.W. 1989. Changes in dental fluorosis following an adjustment to the fluoride concentration of Hong Kong's water supplies. Adv. Dent. Res. 3:154-160.

Evans, R.W., and J.W. Stamm. 1991a. An epidemiologic estimate of the critical period during which human maxillary central incisors are most susceptible to fluorosis. J. Public Health Dent. 51:251-259.

Evans, R.W., and J.W. Stamm. 1991b. Dental fluorosis following downward adjustment of fluoride in drinking water. J. Public Health Dent. 51:91-98.

Faccini, J.M. 1969. Fluoride and bone [review]. Calcif. Tissue Res. 3:1-16.

Farkas, C.S., and E.J. Farkas. 1974. Potential effect of food processing on the fluoride content of infant foods. Sci. Total Environ. 2:399-405.

FDI (Fédération Dentaire Internationale) Commission on Oral Health, Research and Epidemiology. 1982. An epidemiological index of developmental defects of dental enamel (DDE index). Int. Dent. J. 32:159-167.

Featherstone, J.D.B., and C.P. Shields. 1988. A Study of Fluoride Intake in New York State Residents. Final Report. Albany, N.Y.: New York State Health Department.

Fejerskov, O., F. Manji, V. Bælum, and I.J. Möller. 1988. Pp. 51–63 in Dental Fluorosis: A Handbook for Health Workers. Copenhagen: Munksgaard.

Fejerskov, O., F. Manji, and V. Bælum. 1990. The nature and mechanisms of dental fluorosis in man. J. Dent. Res. 69(Spec. Issue): 692–700.

Fejerskov, O., T. Yanagisawa, H. Tohda, M.J. Larsen, K. Josephsen, and H.J. Mosha. 1991. Posteruptive changes in human dental fluorosis—A histological and ultrastructural study. Proc. Finn. Dent. Soc. 87:607–619.

Forrest, J.R., and P.M.C. James. 1965. A blind study of enamel opacities and dental caries prevalence after eight years of fluoridation of water. Br. Dent. J. 119:319–322.

Forsman, B. 1977. Early supply of fluoride and enamel fluorosis. Scand. J. Dent. Res. 85:22–30.

Freni, S.C., and D.W. Gaylor. 1992. International trends in the incidence of bone cancer are not related to drinking water fluoridation. Cancer 70:611–618.

Galagan, D.J. 1953. Climate and controlled fluoridation. J. Am. Dent. Assoc. 47:159–170.

Galagan, D.J., and G.G. Lamson, Jr. 1953. Climate and endemic dental fluorosis. Public Health Rep. 68:497–508.

Galagan, D.J., and J.R. Vermillion. 1957. Determining optimum fluoride concentrations. Public Health Rep. 72:491–493.

Galagan, D.J., J.R. Vermillion, G.A. Nevitt, Z.M. Stadt, and R.E. Dart. 1957. Climate and fluid intake. Public Health Rep. 72:484–490.

Gebhart, E., H. Wagner, and H. Behnsen. 1984. The action of anticlastogens in human lymphocyte cultures and its modification by rat liver S9 mix. I. Studies with AET and sodium fluoride. Mutat. Res. 129:195–206.

Gedalia, I., and L. Shapira. 1989. Effect of prenatal and postnatal fluoride on the human deciduous dentition. A literature review. Adv. Dent. Res. 3:168–176.

Gedalia, I., A. Frumkin, and H. Zukerman. 1964. Effects of estrogen on bone composition in rats at low and high fluoride intake. Endocrinology 75:201-205.

Geever, E.F., N.C. Leone, P. Guser, and J. Lieberman. 1958. Pathologic studies in man after prolonged ingestion of fluoride in drinking water. I. Necropsy findings in a community with a water level of 2.5 ppm. J. Am. Dent. Assoc. 56:499-507.

Gerdes, R.A. 1971. The influence of atmospheric hydrogen fluoride on the frequency of sex-linked recessive lethals and sterility in *Drosophila melanogaster*. Fluoride 4:25-29.

Gocke, E., M.-T. King, K. Eckhardt, and D. Wild. 1981. Mutagenicity of cosmetics ingredients licensed by the European communities. Mutat. Res. 90:91-109.

Goggin, J.E., W. Haddon, Jr., G.S. Hambly, and J.R. Hoveland. 1965. Incidence of femoral fractures in postmenopausal women. Public Health Rep. 80:1005-1012.

Goldman,S.M., M.L. Sievers, and D.W. Templin. 1971. Radiculomyopathy in a southwestern Indian due to skeletal fluorosis. Ariz. Med. 28:675-677.

Gordon, S.L., and S.B. Corbin. 1992. Summary of workshop on drinking water fluoride influence on hip fracture and bone health (National Institutes of Health, April, 10, 1991) [guest editorial]. Osteoporosis Int. 2:109-117.

Grainger, R.M., and C.I. Coburn. 1955. Dental caries of the first molars and the age of children when first consuming naturally fluoridated water. Can. J. Public Health 46:347-354.

Granath, L., J. Widenheim, and D. Birkhed. 1985. Diagnosis of mild enamel fluorosis in permanent maxillary incisors using two scoring systems. Community Dent. Oral Epidemiol. 13:273-276.

Greenberg, S.R. 1986. Response of the renal supporting tissues to chronic fluoride exposure as revealed by a special technique. Urol. Int. 41:91-94.

Griffiths, A.J.F. 1981. Neurospora and environmentally induced aneuploidy. Pp. 187-199 in Short-Term Tests for Chemical Carcinogens, H.F. Stich and R.H.C. San, eds. New York: Springer-Verlag.

Grobler, S.R., C.W. van Wyk, and D. Kotze. 1986. Relationship between enamel fluoride levels, degree of fluorosis and caries experience in communities with a nearly optimal and a high fluoride level in the drinking water. Caries Res. 20:284-288.

Groeneveld, A., A.A.M.J. van Eck, and O. Backer Dirks. 1990. Fluoride in caries prevention: Is the effect pre- or post-eruptive? J. Dent. Res. 69(Spec. Issue):751-755.

Guenter, W. 1979. Fluorine toxicity and laying hen performance [abstract]. Poultry Sci. 58:1063.

Guy, W.S. 1979. Inorganic and organic fluorine in human blood. Pp. 124-147 in Continuing Evaluation of the Use of Fluorides, AAAS Selected Symposium 11, E. Johansen, D.R. Taves, and T.O. Olsen, eds. Boulder, Colo.: Westview Press.

Haimanot, R.T., A. Fekadu, and B. Bushra. 1987. Endemic fluorosis in the Ethiopian Rift Valley. Trop. Geogr. Med. 39:209-217.

Hamdan, M., and W.P. Rock. 1991. The prevalence of enamel mottling on incisor teeth in optimal fluoride and low fluoride communities in England. Community Dent. Health 8:111-119.

Hamilton, I.R. 1990. Biochemical effects of fluoride on oral bacteria. J. Dent. Res. 69(Spec. Issue):660-667.

Hanhijarvi, H. 1975. Inorganic plasma fluoride concentrations and renal excretion in certain physiological and pathological conditions in man. Fluoride 8:198-207.

Hardwick, J.L., J. Teasdale, and G. Bloodworth. 1982. Caries increments over 4 years in children aged 12 at the start of water fluoridation. Br. Dent. J. 153:217-222.

Hargreaves, J.A., G.S. Ingram, and B.J. Wagg. 1972. A gravimetric study of the ingestion of toothpaste by children. Caries Res. 6:237-243.

Harper, R.A., B.A. Flaxman, and D.P. Chopra. 1974. Mitotic response of normal and psoriatic keratinocytes *in vitro* to compounds known to affect intracellular cyclic AMP. J. Invest. Dermatol. 62:384-387.

Haworth, S., T. Lawlor, K. Mortelmans, W. Speck, and E. Zeiger. 1983. *Salmonella* mutagenicity test results for 250 chemicals. Environ. Mutagen. 5(Suppl. 1):1-142.

Hayashi, M., M. Kishi, T. Sofuni, and M. Ishidate, Jr. 1988. Micronucleus tests in mice on 39 food additives and eight miscellaneous chemicals. Food Chem. Toxicol. 26:487-500.

He, W., A. Liu, H. Bao, Y. Wang, and W. Cao. 1983. Effect of sodium fluoride and fluoroacetamide on sister chromatid exchanges and chromosomal aberrations in cultured red muntjac (*Muntjacus muntjak*) cells [in Chinese]. Acta Sci. Circumstantiae 3:94–100.

Heifetz, S.B., W.S. Driscoll, H.S. Horowitz, and A. Kingman. 1988. Prevalence of dental caries and dental fluorosis in areas with optimal and above-optimal water-fluoride concentrations: A 5-year follow-up survey. J. Am. Dent. Assoc. 116:490–495.

Hellström, I. 1960. Fluorine retention following sodium fluoride mouthwashing. Acta Odontol. Scand. 18:263–278.

Hellung-Larsen, P., and H. Klenow. 1969. On the mechanism of inhibition by fluoride ions of the DNA polymerase reaction. Biochim. Biophys. Acta 190:434–441.

Hellwig, E., and J. Klimek. 1985. Caries prevalence and dental fluorosis in German children in areas with different concentrations of fluoride in drinking water supplies. Caries Res. 19:278–283.

Hodge, H.C., and F.A. Smith. 1977. Occupational fluoride exposure. J. Occup. Med. 19:12–39.

Hoffman, D.J., O.H. Pattee, and S.N. Wiemeyer. 1985. Effects of fluoride on screech owl reproduction: Teratological evaluation, growth, and blood chemistry in hatchlings. Toxicol. Lett. 26:19–24.

Holland, R.I. 1979a. Fluoride inhibition of protein and DNA synthesis in cells in vitro. Acta Pharmacol. Toxicol. 45:96–101.

Holland, R.I. 1979b. Fluoride inhibition of DNA synthesis in isolated nuclei from cultured cells. Acta Pharmacol. Toxicol. 45:302–305.

Holm, A.-K., and R. Andersson. 1982. Enamel mineralization disturbances in 12-year-old children with known early exposure to fluorides. Community Dent. Oral Epidemiol. 10:335–339.

Holt, R.D., G.B. Winter, B. Fox, and R. Askew. 1990. Enamel opacities in children whose mothers took part in a dental health education scheme. Community Dent. Oral Epidemiol. 18:74–76.

Hoover, R.N., F.W. McKay, and J.F. Fraumeni, Jr. 1976. Fluoridated drinking water and the occurrence of cancer. J. Natl. Cancer Inst. 57:757–768.

Hoover, R.N., S.S. Devesa, K.P. Cantor, J.H. Lubin, and J.F. Fraumeni, Jr. 1991a. Fluoridation of drinking water and subsequent cancer incidence and mortality. Appendix E in Review of Fluoride Benefits and Risks. Report of the Ad Hoc Subcommittee on Fluoride of the Committee to Coordinate Environmental Health and Related Programs. Washington, D.C.: U.S. Public Health Service.

Hoover, R.N., S. Devesa, K. Cantor, and J.F. Fraumeni, Jr. 1991b. Time trends for bone and joint cancers and osteosarcomas in the Surveillance, Epidemiology and End Results (SEER) Program, National Cancer Institute. Appendix F in Review of Fluoride Benefits and Risks. Report of the Ad Hoc Subcommittee on Fluoride of the Committee to Coordinate Environmental Health and Related Programs. Washington, D.C.: U.S. Public Health Service.

Horowitz, H.S. 1990. The future of water fluoridation and other systemic fluorides. J. Dent. Res. 69(Spec. Issue):760-764.

Horowitz, H.S. 1991. Appropriate uses of fluoride: Considerations for the '90s. Summary. J. Public Health Dent. 51:60-63.

Horowitz, H.S., and S.B. Heifetz. 1967. Effects of prenatal exposure to fluoridation on dental caries. Public Health Rep. 82:297-304.

Horowitz, H.S., W.S. Driscoll, R.J. Meyers, S.B. Heifetz, and A. Kingman. 1984. A new method for assessing the prevalence of dental fluorosis—The Tooth Surface Index of Fluorosis. J. Am. Dent. Assoc. 109:37-41.

Hrudey, S.E., C.L. Soskolne, J. Berkel, and S. Fincham. 1990. Drinking water fluoridation and osteosarcoma. Can. J. Public Health 81:415-416.

IARC (International Agency for Research on Cancer). 1982. Inorganic fluorides. Pp. 235-303 in IARC Monographs on the Evaluation of Carcinogenic Risk of Chemicals to Humans. Some Aromatic Amines, Anthraquinones and Nitroso Compounds, and Inorganic Fluorides Used in Drinking-water and Dental Preparations, Vol. 27. Lyon, France: International Agency for Research on Cancer.

Imai, T., M. Niwa, and M. Ueda. 1983. The effects of fluoride on cell growth of two human cell lines and on DNA and protein synthesis in HeLa cells. Acta Pharmacol. Toxicol. 52:8-11.

Ishidate, M., Jr. 1988. Pp. 381-382 in Data Book of Chromosomal Aberration Test In Vitro, Rev. Ed. Amsterdam: Elsevier.

Ismail, A.I., B.A. Burt, and S.A. Eklund. 1984. The cariogenicity of soft drinks in the United States. J. Am. Dent. Assoc. 109:241-245.

Ismail, A.I., J.-M. Brodeur, M. Kavanagh, G. Boisclair, C. Tessier, and L. Picotte. 1990. Prevalence of dental caries and dental fluorosis in students, 11-17 years of age, in fluoridated and non-fluoridated cities in Quebec. Caries Res. 24:290-297.

Jachimczak, D., and B. Skotarczak. 1978. The effect of fluorine and lead ions on the chromosomes of human leucocytes in vitro. Genet. Polon. 19:353-357.

Jacobsen, S.J., J. Goldberg, T.P. Miles, J.A. Brody, W. Stiers, and A.A. Rimm. 1990. Regional variation in the incidence of hip fracture: U.S. white women aged 65 years and older. JAMA 264:500-502.

Jacobsen, S.J., J. Goldberg, C. Cooper, and S.A. Lockwood. 1992. The association between water fluoridation and hip fracture among white women and men aged 65 years and older: A national ecologic study. Ann. Epidemiol. 2:617-626.

Jacobsen, S.J., W.M. O'Fallon, and L.J. Melton III. 1993. Hip fracture incidence before and after fluoridation of the public water supply, Rochester, Minnesota. Am. J. Public Health 83:743-745.

Jain, S.K., and A.K. Susheela. 1987. Effect of sodium fluoride on antibody formation in rabbits. Environ. Res. 44:117-125.

Johnson, J., Jr., and J.W. Bawden. 1987. The fluoride content of infant formulas available in 1985. Pediatr. Dent. 9:33-37.

Jolly, S.S., B.M. Singh, O.C. Mathur, and K.C. Malhotra. 1968. Epidemiological, clinical, and biochemical study of endemic dental and skeletal fluorosis in Punjab. Br. Med. J. 4:427-429.

Jones, C.A., M.F. Callaham, and E. Huberman. 1988a. Sodium fluoride promotes morphological transformation of Syrian hamster embryo cells. Carcinogenesis 9:2279-2284.

Jones, C.A., E. Huberman, M.F. Callaham, A. Tu, W. Halloween, S. Pallota, A. Sivak, R.A. Lubet, M.D. Avery, R.E. Kouri, J. Spalding, and R.W. Tennant. 1988b. An interlaboratory evaluation of the Syrian hamster embryo cell transformation assay using eighteen coded chemicals. Toxicol. In Vitro 2:103-116.

Kanematsu, N. 1985. Genetic toxicity of biomaterial. 2. DNA damaging effects of sodium fluoride and other fluoride compounds. Jpn. J. Oral Biol. 27:372-374.

Kanisawa, M., and H.A. Schroeder. 1969. Life term studies on the effect of trace elements on spontaneous tumors in mice and rats. Cancer Res. 29:892-895.

Katz, S., and J.C. Muhler. 1968. Prenatal and postnatal fluoride and dental caries experience in deciduous teeth. J. Am. Dent. Assoc. 76:305-311.

Keller, C. 1991. Fluorides in Drinking Water. Paper presented at the Workshop on Drinking Water Fluoride Influence on Hip Fracture and Bone Health, April 10, 1991, Bethesda, Md.

Kidd, E.A.M., A. Thylstrup, O. Fejerskov, and C. Bruun. 1980. Influence of fluoride in surface enamel and degree of dental fluorosis on caries development in vitro. Caries Res. 14:196-202.

Kleerekoper, M., E. Peterson, E. Phillips, D. Nelson, B. Tilley, and A.M. Parfitt. 1989. Continuous sodium fluoride therapy does not reduce vertebral fracture rate in postmenopausal osteoporosis [abstract]. J. Bone Miner. Res. 4(Suppl.1):S376.

Klein, H. 1945. Dental caries experience in relocated children exposed to water containing fluorine. I. Incidence of new caries after 2 years of exposure among previously caries-free permanent teeth. Public Health Rep. 60:1462-1467.

Klein, H. 1946. Dental caries (DMF) experience in relocated children exposed to water containing fluorine. II. J. Am. Dent. Assoc. 33: 1136-1141.

Klein, H. 1975. Dental fluorosis associated with hereditary diabetes insipidus. Oral Surg. Oral Med. Oral Pathol. 40:736-741.

Kleinbaum, D.G., L.L. Kupper, and H. Morganstern. 1982. Information bias. Pp. 220-236 in Epidemiologic Research: Principles and Quantitative Methods. Belmont, Calif.: Lifetime Learning Publications.

Knox, E.G., chairman. 1985. Fluoridation of Water and Cancer: A Review of the Epidemiological Evidence. Report of the Working Party, Department of Health and Social Security. London: Her Majesty's Stationery Office.

Kono, K., Y. Yoshida, M. Watanabe, Y. Tanimura, and T. Hirota. 1984. Urinary fluoride excretion in fluoride exposed workers with diminished renal function. Ind. Health 22:33-40.

Koulourides, T. 1990. Summary of session II: Fluoride and the caries process. J. Dent. Res. 69(Spec. Issue):558.

Kralisz, W., and E. Szymaniak. 1978. Evaluation of the cytogenetic action of sodium fluoride in vitro [in Polish]. Czas. Stomatol. 31: 1109-1113.

Kram, D., E.L. Schneider, L. Singer, and G.R. Martin. 1978. The effects of high and low fluoride diets on the frequencies of sister chromatid exchanges. Mutat. Res. 57:51-55.

Kumar, J.V., E.L. Green, W. Wallace, and T. Carnahan. 1989. Trends in dental fluorosis and dental caries prevalences in Newburgh and Kingston, NY. Am. J. Public Health 79:565-569.

Kuo, H.C., and R.E. Wuthier. 1975. An investigation of fluoride protection against dietary induced osteoporosis in the rat. Clin. Orthop. 110:324-331.

Kuznetsova, L.S. 1969. Effects of industrial factors in superphosphate production on the genitalia of female workers [in Russian]. Gig. Tr. Prof. Zabol. 13(5):21-25.

Lalumandier, J.A. 1992. The prevalence and risk factors of fluorosis among children in a pediatric practice in Asheville, North Carolina [abstract]. J. Public Health Dent. 52:188-189.

Larsen, M.J., A. Richards, and O. Fejerskov. 1985. Development of dental fluorosis according to age at start of fluoride administration. Caries Res. 19:519-527.

Larsen, M.J., E. Kirkegaard, and S. Poulsen. 1987. Patterns of dental fluorosis in a European country in relation to the fluoride concentration of drinking water. J. Dent. Res. 66:10-12.

Larsen, M.J., F. Senderovitz, E. Kirkegaard, S. Poulsen, and O. Fejerskov. 1988. Dental fluorosis in the primary and the permanent dentition in fluoridated areas with consumption of either powdered milk or natural cow's milk. J. Dent. Res. 67:822-825.

Larsen, M.J., E. Kirkegaard, S. Poulsen, and O. Fejerskov. 1989. Dental fluorosis among participants in a non-supervised fluoride tablet program. Community Dent. Oral Epidemiol. 17:204-206.

Lasne, C., Y.-P. Lu, and I. Chouroulinkov. 1988. Transforming activities of sodium fluoride in cultured Syrian hamster embryo and BALB/3T3 cells. Cell Biol. Toxicol. 4:311-324.

LeGeros, R.Z. 1990. Chemical and crystallographic events in the caries process. J. Dent. Res. 69(Spec. Issue):567-574.

Leone, N.C., B.C. Shimkin, F.A. Arnold, C.A. Stevenson, E.R. Zimmermann, P.B. Geiser, and J.E. Lieberman. 1954. Medical aspects of excessive fluoride in a water supply. Public Health Rep. 69:925-936.

Leverett, D.H. 1982. Fluorides and the changing prevalence of dental caries. Science 217:26–30.

Leverett, D. 1986. Prevalence of dental fluorosis in fluoridated and nonfluoridated communities—A preliminary investigation. J. Public Health Dent. 46:184–187.

Levine, R.S. 1976. The action of fluoride in caries prevention: A review of current concepts. Br. Dent. J. 140:9–14.

Levy, S.M., and G. Muchow. 1992. Provider compliance with recommended dietary fluoride supplement protocol. Am. J. Public Health 82:281–283.

Lewis, A., and C.W.M. Wilson. 1985. Fluoride hypersensitivity in mains tap water demonstrated by skin potential changes in guinea pigs. Med. Hypotheses 16:397–402.

Li, Y., A.J. Dunipace, and G.K. Stookey. 1987a. Absence of mutagenic and antimutagenic activities of fluoride in Ames *Salmonella* assays. Mutat. Res. 190:229–236.

Li, Y.M., N.A. Heerema, A.J. Dunipace, and G.K. Stookey. 1987b. Genotoxic effects of fluoride evaluated by sister-chromatid exchange. Mutat. Res. 192:191-201.

Li, Y., A.J. Dunipace, and G.K. Stookey. 1987c. Lack of genotoxic effects of fluoride in the mouse bone-marrow micronucleus test. J. Dent. Res. 66:1687–1690.

Li, Y., A.J. Dunipace, and G.K. Stookey. 1987d. Effects of fluoride on the mouse sperm morphology test. J. Dent. Res. 66:1509–1511.

Li, Y., A.J. Dunipace, and G.K. Stookey. 1988. Genotoxic effects of fluoride: A controversial issue. Mutat. Res. 195:127-136.

Li, Y., W. Zhang, T.W. Noblitt, A.J. Dunipace, and G.K. Stookey. 1989. Genotoxic evaluation of chronic fluoride exposure: Sister-chromatid exchange study. Mutat. Res. 227:159-165.

Lilienfeld, A.M., and D.E. Lilienfeld. 1980. Pp. 213–215 in Foundations of Epidemiology, 2nd Ed. New York: Oxford University Press.

Lim, J.K., G.J. Renaldo, and P. Chapman. 1978. LD_{50} of SnF_2, NaF, and Na_2PO_3F in the mouse compared to the rat. Caries Res. 12:177–179.

Litton Bionetics. 1975. Mutagenic Evaluation of Compound FDA 75-7, 007681-49-4, Sodium Fluoride. Report prepared for the U.S. Food and Drug Administration, Contract 223-74-2104. Kensington, Md.: Litton Bionetics, Inc.

Lynch, C.F. 1984. Fluoride in Drinking Water and State of Iowa Cancer Incidence [Ph.D. thesis]. University of Iowa, Iowa City.

Ma, J., L. Cheng, W. Bai, and H. Wu. 1986. The effects of sodium fluoride on SCEs of mice and on micronucleus of bone marrow of pregnant mice and fetal liver. Hereditas 8:39-41.

MacDonald, D.J., and M.A. Luker. 1980. Fluoride: Interaction with chemical mutagens in *Drosophila*. Mutat. Res. 71:211-218.

Mahoney, M.C., P.C. Nasca, W.S. Burnett, and J.M. Melius. 1991. Bone cancer incidence rates in New York State: Time trends and fluoridated drinking water. Am. J. Public Health 81:475-479.

Mamelle, N., R. Dusan, J.L. Martin, A. Prost, P.J. Meunier, M. Guillaume, A. Gaucher, G. Zeigler, and P. Netter. 1988. Risk-benefit ratio of sodium fluoride treatment in primary vertebral osteoporosis. Lancet II:361-365.

Manji, F., and S. Kapila. 1986a. Fluorides and fluorosis in Kenya. Part I. The occurrence of fluorides. Odont.-Stomatol. Trop. 9:15-20.

Manji, F., and S. Kapila. 1986b. Fluorides and fluorosis in Kenya. Part III. Fluorides, fluorosis, and dental caries. Odont.-Stomatol. Trop. 9:135-139.

Manji, F., V. Bælum, and O. Fejerskov. 1986a. Fluoride, altitude and dental fluorosis. Caries Res. 20:473-480.

Manji, F., V. Bælum, and O. Fejerskov. 1986b. Dental fluorosis in an area of Kenya with 2 ppm fluoride in the drinking water. J. Dent. Res. 65:659-662.

Manji, F., V. Bælum, O. Fejerskov, and W. Gemert. 1986c. Enamel changes in two low-fluoride areas of Kenya. Caries Res. 20:371-380.

Mann, J., M. Tibi, and H.D. Sgan-Cohen. 1987. Fluorosis and caries prevalence in a community drinking above-optimal fluoridated water. Community Dent. Oral Epidemiol. 15:293-295.

Mann, J., W. Mahmoud, M. Ernest, H. Sgan-Cohen, N. Shoshan, and I. Gedalia. 1990. Fluorosis and dental caries in 6-8-year-old children in a 5 ppm fluoride area. Community Dent. Oral Epidemiol. 18:77-79.

Marks, T.A., D. Schellenberg, C.M. Metzler, J. Oostveen, and M.J. Morey. 1984. Effect of dog food containing 460 ppm fluoride on rat reproduction. J. Toxicol. Environ. Health 14:707-714.

Marquis, R.E. 1990. Diminished acid tolerance of plaque bacteria caused by fluoride. J. Dent. Res. 69(Spec. Issue):672-675.

Martin, G.R., K.S. Brown, D.W. Matheson, H. Lebowitz, L. Singer, and R. Ophaug. 1979. Lack of cytogenetic effects in mice or mutations in *Salmonella* receiving sodium fluoride. Mutat. Res. 66:159-167.

Matsuda, A. 1980. Cytogenetic effects of fluoride on human lymphocytes in vitro [in Japanese]. Koku Eisei Gakkai Zasshi 30:312-328.

Matsui, S. 1980. Evaluation of a *Bacillus subtilis* rec-assay for the detection of mutagens which may occur in water environments. Water Res. 14:1613-1619.

Maurer, J.K., M.C. Cheng, B.G. Boysen, and R.L. Anderson. 1990. Two-year carcinogenicity study of sodium fluoride in rats. J. Natl. Cancer Inst. 82:1118-1126.

Maurer, J.K., M.C. Cheng, B.G. Boysen, R.A. Squire, J.D. Strandberg, S.E. Weisbrode, J.L. Seymour, and R.L. Anderson. In press. Confounded carcinogenicity study of sodium fluoride in CD-1 mice. Regul. Toxicol. Pharmacol.

May, D.S., and M.G. Wilson. 1991. Hip Fractures in Relation to Water Fluoridation: An Ecologic Analysis. Paper presented at the Workshop on Drinking Water Fluoride Influence on Hip Fracture and Bone Health, April 10, 1991, Bethesda, Md.

Maylin, G.A., and L. Krook. 1982. Milk production of cows exposed to industrial fluoride pollution. J. Toxicol. Environ. Health 10:473-478.

Mazze, R.I. 1984. Fluorinated anesthetic nephrotoxicity: An update. Can. Anaesth. Soc. J. 31:S16-S22.

McClure, F.J. 1943. Ingestion of fluoride and dental caries: Quantitative relations based on food and water requirements of children one to twelve years old. Am. J. Dis. Child. 66:362-369.

McClure, F.J., H.H. Mitchell, T.S. Hamilton, and C.A. Kinser. 1945. Balances of fluorine ingested from various sources in food and water by five young men. J. Ind. Hyg. Toxicol. 27:159-170.

McGuire, S.M., E.D. Vanable, M.H. McGuire, J.A. Buckwalter, and C.W. Douglass. 1991. Is there a link between fluoridated water and osteosarcoma? J. Am. Dent. Assoc. 122:38-45.

McInnes, P.M., B.D. Richardson, and P.E. Cleaton-Jones. 1982. Comparison of dental fluorosis and caries in primary teeth of pre-school-children living in arid high and low fluoride villages. Community Dent. Oral Epidemiol. 10:182-186.

McKnight-Hanes, M.C., D.H. Leverett, S.M. Adair, and C.P. Shields. 1988. Fluoride content of infant formulas: Soy-based formulas as a potential factor in dental fluorosis. Pediatr. Dent. 10:189–194.

Medvedeva, V.B. 1983. Structure and function of the mucosa of the stomach and duodenum in aluminum smelter workers [abstract]. Gigiena Truda Professions L'nye Zabolevanija 25:8.

Mendelson, D. 1976. Lack of effect of sodium fluoride on a maternal repair system in *Drosophila* oocytes. Mutat. Res. 34:245–250.

Messer, H.H., W.D. Armstrong, and L. Singer. 1973. Influence of fluoride intake on reproduction in mice. J. Nutr. 103:1319–1326.

Milsom, K., and C.M. Mitropoulos. 1990. Enamel defects in 8-year-old children in fluoridated and non-fluoridated parts of Cheshire. Caries Res. 24:286–289.

Mircevova, L., L. Viktora, and E. Hermanova. 1984. Inhibition of phagocytes of polymorphonuclear leucocytes by adenosine and $HoCl_3$ in vitro. Med. Biol. 62:326–330.

Mitchell, B., and R. Gerdes. 1973. Mutagenic effects of sodium and stannous fluoride upon *Drosophila melanogaster*. Fluoride 6(2):113–117.

Mitchell, H.H., and M. Edman. 1952. The fluorine problem in live-stock feeding. Nutr. Abst. Rev. 21:787–804.

Mizuguchi, J., N. Utsunomiya, M. Nakanishi, Y. Arata, and H. Fuka-zawa. 1989. Differential sensitivity of anti-IgM-induced and NaF-induced inositol phospholipid metabolism to serine protease inhibitors in BAL17 B lymphoma cells. Biochem. J. 263:641–646.

Modly, C.E., and J.W. Burnett. 1987. Dermatologic manifestations of fluoride exposure. Cutis 40:89–90.

Mohamed, A.H., and M.E. Chandler. 1982. Cytological effects of sodium fluoride on mice. Fluoride 15(3):110–118.

Møller, I.J., J.J. Pindborg, I. Gedalia, and B. Roed-Petersen. 1970. The prevalence of dental fluorosis in the people of Uganda. Arch. Oral Biol. 15:213–225.

Mukherjee, R.N., and F.H. Sobels. 1968. The effects of sodium fluoride and iodoacetamide on mutation induction by x-irradiation in mature spermatozoa of *Drosophila*. Mutat. Res. 6:217–225.

Myers, H.M. 1978. Fluorides and Dental Fluorosis. Monographs in Oral Science, Vol. 7. Basel, Switzerland: Karger.

Myers, H.M. 1983. Dose-response relationship between water fluoride levels and the category of questionable dental fluorosis. Community Dent. Oral Epidemiol. 11:109-112.

National Health and Medical Research Council. 1985. Report of Working Party on fluorides in the control of dental caries. Aust. Dent. J. 30:433-442.

Nair, K.R., and F. Manji. 1982. Endemic fluorosis in deciduous dentition: A study of 1276 children in typically high fluoride area (Kiambu) in Kenya. Odontostomatol. Trop. 5:177-184.

Naylor, M.N., and R.F. Wilson. 1967. The effect of fluoridated drinking water on the physical properties of the rat femur. J. Physiol. 189:55P.

Nelson, D.G.A., G.E. Coote, I.C. Vickridge, and G. Suckling. 1989. Proton microprobe determination of fluorine profiles in the enamel and dentine of erupting incisors from sheep given low and high daily doses of fluoride. Arch. Oral Biol. 34:419-429.

Nikiforova, V.Y. 1982. Mechanism of the mutagenic action of fluoride. Cytol. Genet. (Engl. Transl.) 16:40-42.

Nopakun, J., and H.H. Messer. 1989. Mechanisms of fluoride transfer across the small intestine in vitro [abstract]. J. Dent. Res. 68(Spec. Issue):287.

NRC (National Research Council). 1977. Inorganic solutes. Pp. 205-488 in Drinking Water and Health. Washington, D.C.: National Research Council.

NRC (National Research Council). 1989. Recommended Dietary Allowances, 10th Ed. Washington, D.C.: National Research Council.

NTP (National Toxicology Program). 1990. Toxicology and Carcino-genesis Studies of Sodium Fluoride in F344/N Rats and B6C3F$_1$ Mice. Technical Report Series No. 393. NIH Publ. No. 91-2848. Research Triangle Park, N.C.: National Institute of Environmental Health Sciences.

Okada, K., and E.J. Brown. 1988. Sodium fluoride reveals multiple pathways for regulation of surface expression of the C3b/C4b receptor (CR1) on human polymorphonuclear leukocytes. J. Immunol. 140: 878-884.

Olsson, B. 1979. Dental findings in high-fluoride areas in Ethiopia. Community Dent. Oral Epidemiol. 7:51-56.

O'Mullane, D.M., and J. Clarkson. 1990. The risk of fluorosis in a fluoridated community: A critique of the Toronto study [abstract]. Community Dent. Health 7:316.

Ophaug, R.H., L. Singer, and B.F. Harland. 1980a. Estimated fluoride intake of average two-year-old children in four dietary regions of the United States. J. Dent. Res. 59:777–781.

Ophaug, R.H., L. Singer, and B.F. Harland. 1980b. Estimated fluoride intake of 6-month-old infants in four dietary regions of the United States. Am. J. Clin. Nutr. 33:324–327.

Ophaug, R.H., L. Singer, and B.F. Harland. 1985. Dietary fluoride intake of 6-month and 2-year-old children in four dietary regions of the United States. Am. J. Clin. Nutr. 42:701–707.

O'Shea, J.J., K.B. Urdahl, H.T. Luong, T.M. Chused, L.E. Samelson, and R.D. Klausner. 1987. Aluminum fluoride induces phosphatidyl-inositol turnover, elevation of cytoplasmic free calcium, and phosphorylation of the T cell antigen receptor in murine T cells. J. Immunol. 139:3463–3469.

Osuji, O.O., J.L. Leake, M.L. Chipman, G. Nikiforuk, D. Locker, and N. Levine. 1988. Risk factors for dental fluorosis in a fluoridated community. J. Dent. Res. 67:1488–1492.

Pang, D.T.Y., C.L. Phillips, and J.W. Bawden. 1992. Fluoride intake from beverage consumption in a sample of North Carolina children. J. Dent. Res. 71:1382–1388.

Parkins, F.M. 1972. Retention of fluoride with chewable tablets and mouth rinses. J. Dent. Res. 51:1346–1349.

Pashley, D.H., N.B. Allison, R.P. Easmann, R.V. McKinney, Jr., J.A. Horner, and G.M. Whitford. 1984. The effects of fluoride on the gastric mucosa of the rat. J. Oral Pathol. 13:535–545.

Pati, P.C., and S.P. Bhunya. 1987. Genotoxic effect of an environmental pollutant, sodium fluoride, in mammalian in vivo test system. Caryologia 40:79–87.

Pattee, O.H., S.N. Wiemeyer, and D.M. Swineford. 1988. Effects of dietary fluoride on reproduction in Eastern screech owls. Arch. Environ. Contam. Toxicol. 17:213–218.

Pendrys, D.G. 1990. The fluorosis risk index: A method for investigating risk factors. J. Public Health Dent. 50:291–298.

Pendrys, D.G., and R.V. Katz. 1989. Risk of enamel fluorosis associated with fluoride supplementation, infant formula, and fluoride dentifrice use. Am. J. Epidemiol. 130:1199-1208.

Pendrys, D.G., and D.E. Morse. 1990. Use of fluoride supplementation by children living in fluoridated communities. J. Dent. Child. 57:343-347.

Pendrys, D.G., and J.W. Stamm. 1990. Relationship of total fluoride intake to beneficial effects and enamel fluorosis. J. Dent. Res. 69 (Spec. Issue):529-538.

Phillips, P.H., A.R. Lamb, E.B. Hart, and G. Bohstedt. 1933. Studies on fluorine in the nutrition of the rat. II. Its influence upon reproduction. Am. J. Physiol. 106:356-364.

Phillips, P.H., E.B. Hart, and G. Bohstedt. 1934. Chronic toxicosis in dairy cows due to ingestion of fluorine. Wisc. Agr. Exp. Station Res. Bull. 123:1-30.

PHS (U.S. Public Health Service). 1962. Public Health Service Drinking Water Standards, Revised 1962. PHS Publ. No. 956. Washington, D.C.: U.S. Government Printing Office.

PHS (U.S. Public Health Service). 1991. Review of Fluoride Benefits and Risks. Report of the Ad Hoc Subcommittee on Fluoride of the Committee to Coordinate Environmental Health and Related Programs. Washington D.C.: U.S. Public Health Service.

Rahn, K.A., R. Vanderby, Jr., S.S. Kohles, B.J. Kiratli, R.J. Thielke, A.B. Clay, and J.W. Suttie. 1991. Mechanical effects of sodium fluoride on bovine cortical bone. Clin. Biomech. 6:185-189.

Rall, D.P. 1991. Carcinogens and human health: Part 2 [letter]. Science 251:10-12.

Razak, I.A., and R.J. Latifah. 1988. Unusual hypersensitivity reaction to stannous fluoride. Ann. Dent. 47:37-39.

Rich, C., and E. Feist. 1970. The action of fluoride on bone. Pp. 70-87 in Fluoride in Medicine, T.C. Vischer, ed. Bern, Switzerland: Hans Huber.

Rich, C., J. Ensink, and Peter Ivanovich. 1964. The effects of sodium fluoride on calcium metabolism of subjects with metabolic bone diseases. J. Clin. Invest. 43:545-456.

Richards, A. 1990. Nature and mechanisms of dental fluorosis in animals. J. Dent. Res. 69(Spec. Issue):701-705.

Richards, A., J. Kragstrup, K. Josephsen, and O. Fejerskov. 1986. Dental fluorosis developed in post-secretory enamel. J. Dent. Res. 65:1406-1409.

Richards, A., O. Fejerskov, and V. Bælum. 1989. Enamel fluoride in relation to severity of human dental fluorosis. Adv. Dent. Res. 3:147-153.

Richards, L.F., W.W. Westmoreland, M. Tashiro, C.H. McKay, and J.T. Morrison. 1967. Determining optimum fluoride levels for community water supplies in relation to temperature. J. Am. Dent. Assoc. 74:389-397.

Richmond, V.L. 1985. Thirty years of fluoridation: A review. Am. J. Clin. Nutr. 41:129-138.

Riggins, R.S., F. Zeman, and D. Moon. 1974. The effects of sodium fluoride on bone breaking strength. Calcif. Tissue Res. 14:283-289.

Riggs, B.L., S.F. Hodgson, W.M. O'Fallon, E.Y.S. Chao, H.W. Wahner, J.M. Muhs, S.L. Cedel, and L.J. Melton III. 1990. Effect of fluoride treatment on the fracture rate in postmenopausal women with osteoporosis. N. Engl. J. Med. 322:802-809.

Riordan, P.J., and J.A. Banks. 1991. Dental fluorosis and fluoride exposure in Western Australia. J. Dent. Res. 70:1022-1028.

Romanus, B. 1974. Physical properties and chemical content of canine femoral cortical bone in nutritional osteopenia: Its reversibility. Acta Orthop. Scand. Suppl. 155:1-101.

Rosen, D., I. Gedalia, J. Anaise, A. Simkin, and M. Arcan. 1975. The effect of fluoride alone or fluoride followed by calcium and vitamin D on disuse osteoporosis of the rat tail vertebrae. Calcif. Tissue Res. 19:9-15.

Rosen, S., J.I. Frea, and S.M. Hsu. 1978. Effect of fluoride-resistant microorganisms on dental caries. J. Dent. Res. 57:180.

Rozier, R.G. 1991. Reaction paper: Appropriate uses of fluoride—Considerations for the '90s. J. Public Health Dent. 51:56-59.

Russell, A.L. 1961. The differential diagnosis of fluoride and non-fluoride enamel opacities. J. Public Health Dent. 21:143-146.

Russell, A.L. 1962. Dental fluorosis in Grand Rapids during the seventeenth year of fluoridation. J. Am. Dent. Assoc. 65:608-612.

Russell, A.L., and P.M. Hamilton. 1961. Dental caries in permanent first molars after eight years of fluoridation. Arch. Oral Biol. 6(Spec. Suppl.):50-57.

San Filippo, F.A., and G.C. Battistone. 1971. The fluoride content of a representative diet of the young male adult. Clin. Chim. Acta 31:453–457.

Sato, T., K. Kitada, S. Onoue, T. Nagano, M. Hoshiai, K. Osozawa, and M. Niwa. 1989. Effect of fluoride on human peripheral lymphocytes in vitro: Chromosome observations and biochemical study [in Japanese]. Koku Eisei Gakkai Zasshi 39:632–633.

Sauerbrunn, B.J.L., C.M. Ryan, and J.F. Shaw. 1965. Chronic fluoride intoxication with fluorotic radiculomyelopathy. Ann. Intern. Med. 63:1074–1078.

Saville, P.D. 1967. Water fluoridation: Effect on bone fragility and skeletal calcium content in the rat. J. Nutr. 91:353–357.

Schellenberg, D., T.A. Marks, C.M. Metzler, J.A. Oostveen, and M.J. Morey. 1990. Lack of effect of fluoride on reproductive performance and development in Shetland sheepdogs. Vet. Hum. Toxicol. 32:309– 314; erratum 32:527.

Schenker, M., J. Beaumont, B. Eskenazi, E. Gold, K. Hammond, B. Lasley, S. McCurdy, S. Samuels, and S. Swan. 1992. Final Report to the Semiconductor Industry Association: Epidemiologic Study of Reproductive and Other Health Effects Among Workers Employed in the Manufacture of Semiconductors. Davis, Ca.: University of California at Davis.

Schiffl, H.H., and U. Binswanger. 1980. Human urinary fluoride excretion as influenced by renal functional impairment. Nephron 26:69–72.

Schiffl, H., and U. Binswanger. 1982. Renal handling of fluoride in healthy man. Renal Physiol. 5:192–195.

Schlesinger, E.R., D.E. Overton, H.C. Chase, and K.T. Cantwell. 1956. Newburgh-Kingston caries—fluorine study. XIII: Pediatric findings after ten years. J. Am. Dent. Assoc. 52:296–306.

Scott, D., and S.A. Roberts. 1987. Extrapolation from in vitro tests to human risk: Experience with sodium fluoride clastogenicity. Mutat. Res. 189:47–58.

Segreto, V.A., E.M. Collins, D. Camann, and C.T. Smith. 1984. A current study of mottled enamel in Texas. J. Am. Dent. Assoc. 108:56–59.

Shambaugh, G.E., Jr., and V.S. Sundar. 1969. Experiments and experiences with sodium fluoride for inactivation of the otosclerotic lesion. Laryngoscope 79:1754-1764.

Sharma, R.P., P.T. Blotter, and J.L. Shupe. 1977. Fluoride accumulation in bone and the effect on their physical properties in guinea pigs given different levels of fluoridated water. Clin. Toxicol. 11:329-339.

Shen, Y.W., and D.R. Taves. 1974. Fluoride concentrations in the human placenta and maternal and cord blood. Am. J. Obstet. Gynecol. 119:205-207.

Silverstone, L.M. 1977. Remineralization phenomena. Caries Res. 11(Suppl. 1):59-84.

Singer, L., B.A. Jarvey, P. Venkateswarlu, and W.D. Armstrong. 1970. Fluoride in plaque. J. Dent. Res. 49:455.

Singer, L., R.H. Ophaug, and B.F. Harland. 1980. Fluoride intakes of young male adults in the United States. Am. J. Clin. Nutr. 33:328-332.

Singh, A., and S.S. Jolly. 1970. Chronic toxic effects on the skeletal system. Pp. 238-249 in Fluorides and Human Health. Geneva: World Health Organization.

Skare, J.A., T.K. Wong, B.L.B. Evans, and D.B. Cody. 1986a. DNA-repair studies with sodium fluoride: Comparative evaluation using density gradient ultracentrifugation and autoradiography. Mutat. Res. 172:77-87.

Skare, J.A., K.R. Schrotel, and G.A. Nixon. 1986b. Lack of DNA-strand breaks in rat testicular cells after in vivo treatment with sodium fluoride. Mutat. Res. 170:85-92.

Slamenová, D., A. Gábelová, and K. Ruppová. 1992. Cytotoxicity and genotoxicity testing of sodium fluoride on Chinese hamster V79 cells and human EUE cells. Mutat. Res. 279:109-115.

Smith, F.A., and H.C. Hodge. 1979. Airborne fluorides and man. Crit. Rev. Environ. Control 9:1-25.

Sowers, M.F.R., M.K. Clark, M.L. Jannausch, and R.B. Wallace. 1991. A prospective study of bone mineral content and fracture in communities with differential fluoride exposure. Am. J. Epidemiol. 133:649-660.

Spak, C.J., L.I. Hardell, and P. de Chateau. 1983. Fluoride in human milk. Acta Paediatr. Scand. 72:699-701.

Spak, C.J., U. Berg, and J. Ekstrand. 1985. Renal clearance of fluoride in children and adolescents. Pediatrics 75:575-579.

Srivastava, S.K., E. Gillerman, and M.J. Modak. 1981. The artifactual nature of fluoride inhibition of reverse transcriptase and associated ribonuclease H. Biochem. Biophys. Res. Commun. 101:183-188.

Stephen, K.W., D.R. McCall, and W.H. Gilmour. 1991. Incisor enamel mottling prevalence in child cohorts which had or had not taken fluoride supplements from 0-12 years of age. Proc. Finn. Dent. Soc. 87:595-605.

Stevenson, C.A., and A.R. Watson. 1957. Fluoride osteosclerosis. Am. J. Roentgenol. Radium Ther. Nucl. Med. 78:13-18.

Subbareddy, V.V., and A. Tewari. 1985. Enamel mottling at different levels of fluoride in drinking water: In an endemic area. J. Indian Dent. Assoc. 57:205-212.

Suckling, G.W., and E.I. Pearce. 1984. Developmental defects of enamel in a group of New Zealand children: Their prevalence and some associated etiological factors. Community Dent. Oral Epidemiol. 12:177-184.

Suckling, G., D.C. Thurley, and D.G.A. Nelson. 1988. The macroscopic and scanning electron-microscopic appearance and microhardness of the enamel, and the related histological changes in the enamel organ of erupting sheep incisors resulting from a prolonged low daily dose of fluoride. Arch. Oral Biol. 33:361-373.

Suttie, J.W., J.R. Carlson, and E.C. Faltin. 1972. Effects of alternating periods of high- and low-fluoride ingestion on dairy cattle. J. Dairy Sci. 55:790-804.

Szpunar, S.M., and B.A. Burt. 1987. Trends in the prevalence of dental fluorosis in the United States: A review. J. Public Health Dent. 47:71-79.

Szpunar, S.M., and B.A. Burt. 1988. Dental caries, fluorosis, and fluoride exposure in Michigan schoolchildren. J. Dent. Res. 67:802-806.

Szpunar, S.M., and B.A. Burt. 1992. Evaluation of appropriate use of dietary fluoride supplements in the U.S. Community Dent. Oral Epidemiol. 20:148-154.

Takanaka, K., and P.J. O'Brien. 1985. Proton release by polymorphonuclear leukocytes during phagocytosis or activation by digitonin or fluoride. Biochem. Int. 11:127-136.

Tannenbaum, A., and H. Silverstone. 1949. Effect of low environmental temperature, dinitrophenol, or sodium fluoride on the formation of tumors in mice. Cancer Res. 9:403–410.

Tao, S., and J.W. Suttie. 1976. Evidence for a lack of an effect of dietary fluoride level on reproduction in mice. J. Nutr. 106:1115–1122.

Tatevossian, A. 1990. Fluoride in dental plaque and its effects. J. Dent. Res. 69(Spec. Issue):645–652.

Taves, D.R. 1968. Determination of submicromolar concentrations of fluoride in biological samples. Talanta 15:1015–1023.

Taves, D.R. 1983. Dietary intake of fluoride ashed (total fluoride) v. unashed (inorganic fluoride) analysis of individual foods. Br. J. Nutr. 49:295–301.

Taylor, A. 1954. Sodium fluoride in the drinking water of mice. Dent. Dig. 60:170–172.

Taylor, A., and N.C. Taylor. 1965. Effect of sodium fluoride on tumor growth. Proc. Soc. Exp. Biol. Med. 119:252–255.

Taylor, J.M., J.K. Scott, E.A. Maynard, F.A. Smith, and H.C. Hodge. 1961. Toxic effects of fluoride on the rat kidney. I. Acute injury from single large doses. Toxicol. Appl. Pharmacol. 3:278–289.

Thomson, E.J., F.M. Kilanowski, and P.E. Perry. 1985. The effect of fluoride on chromosome aberration and sister-chromatid exchange frequencies in cultured human lymphocytes. Mutat. Res. 144:89–92.

Thylstrup, A. 1978. Distribution of dental fluorosis in the primary dentition. Community Dent. Oral Epidemiol. 6:329–337.

Thylstrup, A. 1983. Posteruptive development of isolated and confluent pits in fluorosed enamel in a 6-year-old girl. Scand. J. Dent. Res. 91:243–246.

Thylstrup, A. 1990. Clinical evidence of the role of pre-eruptive fluoride in caries prevention. J. Dent. Res. 69(Spec. Issue):742–750.

Thylstrup, A., and O. Fejerskov. 1978. Clinical appearance of dental fluorosis in permanent teeth in relation to histologic changes. Community Dent. Oral Epidemiol. 6:315–328.

Thylstrup, A., O. Fejerskov, C. Bruun, and J. Kann. 1979. Enamel changes and dental caries in 7-year-old children given fluoride tablets from shortly after birth. Caries Res. 13:265–276.

Tokar, V.I., and O.N. Savchenko. 1977. Effect of inorganic fluorine compounds on the functional condition of the hypophysis-testes system [in Russian]. Probl. Endokrinol. 23:104–107.

Tong, C.C., C.A. McQueen, S. Ved Brat, and G.M. Williams. 1988. The lack of genotoxicity of sodium fluoride in a battery of cellular tests. Cell Biol. Toxicol. 4:173–186.

Tsutsui, T., N. Suzuki, and H. Ohmori. 1984a. Sodium fluoride-induced morphological and neoplastic transformation, chromosome aberrations, sister chromatid exchanges, and unscheduled DNA synthesis in cultured Syrian hamster embryo cells. Cancer Res. 44:938–941.

Tsutsui, T., N. Suzuki, M. Ohmori, and H. Maizumi. 1984b. Cytotoxicity, chromosome aberrations and unscheduled DNA synthesis in cultured human diploid fibroblasts induced by sodium fluoride. Mutat. Res. 139:193–198.

Tsutsui, T., K. Ide, and H. Maizumi. 1984c. Induction of unscheduled DNA synthesis in cultured human oral keratinocytes by sodium fluoride. Mutat. Res. 140:43–48.

Turner, C.H., M.P. Akhter, and R.P. Heaney. 1992. The effects of fluoridated water on bone strength. J. Orthop. Res. 10:581–587.

van Loveren, C. 1990. The antimicrobial action of fluoride and its role in caries inhibition. J. Dent. Res. 69(Spec. Issue):676–681.

van Rensburg, S.W.J., and W.H. de Vos. 1966. The influence of excess fluorine intake in the drinking water on reproductive efficiency in bovines. Onderstepoort J. Vet. Res. 33:185–194.

Venkateswarlu, P. 1990. Evaluation of analytical methods for fluorine in biological and related materials. J. Dent. Res. 69(Spec. Issue): 514–521.

Vogel, E. 1973. Strong antimutagenic effects of fluoride on mutation induction by trenimon and 1-phenyl-3,3-dimethyltriazene in *Drosophila melanogaster*. Mutat. Res. 20:339–352.

Voroshilin, S.I., E.G. Plotko, E.Z. Gatiyatullina, and E.A. Gileva. 1975. Cytogenetic effect of inorganic fluorine compounds on human and animal cells in vivo and in vitro. Sov. Genet. (Engl. Transl.) 9:492–496.

Waldbott, G.L. 1962. Fluoride in clinical medicine. Int. Arch. Allergy Appl. Immunol. 20(Suppl. 1):29.

Waldbott, G.L., and A.W. Burgstahler. 1978. Fluoridation. The Great Dilemma. Lawrence, Kan.: Coronado Press.

Waldbott, G.L., and V.A. Cecilioni. 1969. Neighborhood fluorosis. Fluoride 2:206-213.

Waldbott, G.L., and S. Steinegger. 1973. New observations on "Chizzola maculae." Proc. Third Int. Clean Air Congress. Dusseldorf, Germany.

Walvekar, S.V., and B.A. Qureshi. 1982. Endemic fluorosis and partial defluoridation of water supplies—A public health concern in Kenya. Community Dent. Oral Epidemiol. 10:156-160.

Waterhouse, C., D. Taves, and A. Munzer. 1980. Serum inorganic fluoride: Changes related to previous fluoride intake, renal function and bone resorption. Clin. Sci. 58:145-152.

Weatherell, J.A., D. Deutsch, C. Robinson, and A.S. Hallsworth. 1977. Assimilation of fluoride by enamel throughout the life of the tooth. Caries Res. 11(Suppl. 1):85-115.

Weeks, K.J. 1990. Enamel mottling in a non-fluoride community since the advent of fluoride toothpastes. Br. Dent. J. 169:258-260.

Wefel, J.S., G. Maharry, M.E. Jensen, P. Hayes, and B.H. Clarkson. 1986. In vivo demineralization and remineralization of enamel and root surfaces. Pp. 181-190 in Factors Relating to Demineralisation and Remineralisation of the Teeth, S.A. Leach, ed. Oxford, U.K.: IRL Press.

Wei, S.H., and M.J. Kanellis. 1983. Fluoride retention after sodium fluoride mouthrinsing by pre-school children. J. Am. Dent. Assoc. 106:626-629.

Wenzel, A., A. Thylstrup, B. Melsen, and O. Fejerskov. 1982. The relationship between water-borne fluoride, dental fluorosis, and skeletal development in 11-15 year old Tanzanian girls. Arch. Oral Biol. 27:1007-1011.

White, D.J., and G.H. Nancollas. 1990. Physical and chemical considerations of the role of firmly and loosely bound fluoride in caries prevention. J. Dent. Res. 69(Spec. Issue):587-594.

Whitford, G.M. 1989. The Metabolism and Toxicity of Fluoride. Monographs in Oral Science No. 13, H.M. Myers, ed. Basel, Switzerland: Karger.

Whitford, G.M. 1990. The physiological and toxicological characteristics of fluoride. J. Dent. Res. 69(Spec. Issue):539-549, 556-557.

Whitford, G.M. 1991. Fluoride, calcium, and phosphorus metabolism in the rat: Comparison of 'natural ingredient' with semipurified diets. Arch. Oral Biol. 36:291-297.

Whitford, G.M., and D.H. Pashley. 1984. Fluoride absorption: The influence of gastric acidity. Calcif. Tissue Int. 36:302-307.

Whitford, G.M., and D.H. Pashley. 1991. Fluoride reabsorption by nonionic diffusion in the distal nephron of the dog. Proc. Soc. Exp. Biol. Med. 196:178-183.

Whitford, G.M., and K.E. Reynolds. 1979. Plasma and developing enamel fluoride concentrations during chronic acid-base disturbances. J. Dent. Res. 58:2058-2065.

Whitford, G.M., and J.L. Williams. 1986. Fluoride absorption: Independence from plasma fluoride levels. Proc. Soc. Exp. Biol. Med. 181:550-554.

Whitford, G.M., D.H. Pashley, and G.I. Stringer. 1976. Fluoride renal clearance: A pH-dependent event. Am. J. Physiol. 230:527-532.

Whitford, G.M., D.H. Pashley, and K.E. Reynolds. 1979. Fluoride tissue distribution: Short-term kinetics. Am. J. Physiol. 236:F141-F148.

Whitford, G.M., D.W. Allmann, and A.R. Shahed. 1987. Topical fluorides: Effects on physiologic and biochemical processes. J. Dent. Res. 66:1072-1078.

Williams, J.E., and J.D. Zwemer. 1990. Community water fluoride levels, preschool dietary patterns, and the occurrence of fluoride enamel opacities. J. Public Health Dent. 50:276-281.

Wolinsky, I., A. Simkin, and K. Guggenheim. 1972. Effects of fluoride on metabolism and mechanical properties of rat bone. Am. J. Physiol. 223:46-50.

Wöltgens, J.H.M., E.J. Etty, W.M.D. Nieuwland, and D.M. Lyaruu. 1989. Use of fluoride by young children and prevalence of mottled enamel. Adv. Dent. Res. 3:177-182.

Woolfolk, M.W., B.W. Faja, and R.A. Bagramian. 1989. Relation of sources of systemic fluoride to prevalence of dental fluorosis. J. Public Health Dent. 49:78-82.

Workshop Report. 1992. Changing patterns of fluoride intake. Workshop. Chapel Hill, April 23-25, 1991. J. Dent. Res. 71:1214-1227.

Yanagisawa, T., S. Takum, and O. Fejerskov. 1989. Ultrastructure and composition of enamel in human dental fluorosis. Adv. Dent. Res. 3:203–210.

Yiamouyiannis, J., and D. Burk. 1977. Fluoridation and cancer: Age-dependence of cancer mortality related to artificial fluoridation. Fluoride10:102–125.

APPENDIX 1

Criteria for Dean's Index, TF Index, and TSIF

TABLE A-1 Criteria for Dean's Fluorosis Index

Diagnosis	Criteria
Normal	The enamel represents the usually translucent semivitriform type of structure. The surface is smooth, glossy, and usually a pale creamy white color.
Questionable	The enamel discloses slight aberrations from the translucency of normal enamel, ranging from a few white flecks to occasional white spots. This classification is utilized in those instances where a definite diagnosis of the mildest form of fluorosis is not warranted and a classification of "normal" is not justified.
Very mild	Small, opaque, paper white area scattered irregularly over the tooth but not involving as much as approximately 25% of the tooth surface. Frequently included in this classification are teeth showing no more than about 1-2 mm of white opacity at the tip of the summit of the cusps of the bicuspids or second molars.
Mild	The white opaque areas in the enamel of the teeth are more extensive but do not involve as much as 50% of the tooth.
Moderate	All enamel surfaces of the teeth are affected, and surfaces subject to attrition show marked wear. Brown stain is frequently a disfiguring feature.
Severe	Includes teeth formerly classified as "moderately severe and severe." All enamel surfaces are affected and hypoplasia is so marked that the general form of the tooth may be altered. The major diagnostic sign of this classification is the discrete or confluent pitting. Brown stains are widespread and teeth often present a corroded appearance.

Source: Dean, 1942. Reprinted with permission; copyright 1942, American Association for the Advancement of Science.

TABLE A-2 Clinical Criteria and Scoring System for the Tooth
Surface Index of Fluorosis

Score	Criteria
0	Enamel shows no evidence of fluorosis.
1	Enamel shows definite evidence of fluorosis, namely, areas with parchment-white color that total less than one-third of the visible enamel surface. This category includes fluorosis confined only to incisal edges of anterior teeth and cusp tips of posterior teeth ("snowcapping").
2	Parchment-white fluorosis totals at least one-third of the visible surface, but less than two-thirds.
3	Parchment-white fluorosis totals at least two-thirds of the visible surface.
4	Enamel shows staining in conjunction with any of the preceding levels of fluorosis. Staining is defined as an area of definite discoloration that may range from light to very dark brown.
5	Discrete pitting of the enamel exists, unaccompanied by evidence of staining of intact enamel. A pit is defined as a definite physical defect in the enamel surface with a rough floor that is surrounded by a wall of intact enamel. The pitted area is usually stained or differs in color from the surrounding enamel.
6	Both discrete pitting and staining of the intact enamel exist.
7	Confluent pitting of the enamel surface exists. Large areas of enamel may be missing and the anatomy of the tooth may be altered. Dark-brown stain is usually present.

Source: Horowitz et al., 1984. Reprinted with permission;
copyright 1984, American Dental Association.

TABLE A-3 Clinical Criteria and Scoring for the TF Index

Score	Criteria
0	Normal translucency of enamel remains after prolonged air-drying.
1	Narrow white lines corresponding to the perikymata.
2	*Smooth surfaces*: More pronounced lines of opacity that follow the perikymata. Occasionally confluence of adjacent lines. *Occlusal surfaces*: Scattered areas of opacity < 2 mm in diameter and pronounced opacity of cuspal ridges.
3	*Smooth surfaces*: Merging and irregular cloudy areas of opacity. Accentuated drawing of perikymata often visible between opacities. *Occlusal surfaces*: Confluent areas of marked opacity. Worn areas appear almost normal but usually circumscribed by a rim of opaque enamel.
4	*Smooth surfaces*: The entire surface exhibits marked opacity or appears chalky white. Parts of surface exposed to attrition appear less affected. *Occlusal surfaces*: Entire surface exhibits marked opacity. Attrition is often pronounced shortly after eruption.
5	*Smooth surfaces and occlusal surfaces*: Entire surface displays marked opacity with focal loss of outermost enamel (pits) < 2 mm in diameter.
6	*Smooth surfaces*: Pits are regularly arranged in horizontal bands < 2 mm in vertical extension. *Occlusal surfaces*: Confluent areas < 3 mm in diameter exhibit loss of enamel. Marked attrition.
7	*Smooth surfaces*: Loss of outermost enamel in irregular areas involving < 1/2 of entire surface. *Occlusal surfaces*: Changes in the morphology caused by merging pits and marked attrition.
8	*Smooth and occlusal surfaces*: Loss of outermost enamel involving > 1/2 of surface.
9	*Smooth and occlusal surfaces*: Loss of main part of enamel with change in anatomic appearance of surface. Cervical rim of almost unaffected enamel is often noted.

Source: Thylstrup and Fejerskov, 1978. Reprinted with permission from *Community Dentistry and Oral Epidemiology*; copyright 1978.

APPENDIX 2

Letter to AFIP

NATIONAL RESEARCH COUNCIL

BOARD ON ENVIRONMENTAL STUDIES
AND TOXICOLOGY

2101 Constitution Avenue   Washington, D.C. 20418

COMMITTEE ON TOXICOLOGY

TEL: (202) 334-2616
FAX: (202) 334-1393

July 24, 1992

Colonel John M. Pletcher
Department of Veterinary Pathology
Armed Forces Institute of Pathology
Washington, DC 20306-6000

Dear Col. Pletcher:

The National Research Council's Committee on Toxicology has organized the Subcommittee on Risk Assessment of Ingested Fluoride. This study was requested by the U.S. Environmental Protection Agency to determine if the current drinking water standard for fluoride (4 mg/L) is appropriate.

At its second meeting on July 13, 1992, in Aspen, CO, the subcommittee recommended the review of Procter and Gamble's mouse fluoride carcinogenicity study by the Armed Forces Institute of Pathology (AFIP) for the following:

- What is the proper terminology for these lesions?

- Should the osteomas be considered neoplasms?

- Is there a hyperostosis/osteoma continuum?

- Do the osteomas have potential for malignant change?

- Would these lesions regress if the stimulus were removed?

- How often are bone neoplasms in animals multicentric?

- Is there a human counterpart for these lesions?

- Of those people involved, there is general knowledge of a contaminating virus in this mouse study. What evidence is available to confirm it?

We have requested Procter and Gamble to submit mouse slides to AFIP for its independent review. The final meeting of the subcommittee is scheduled for October 16, 1992, in Washington, DC. Therefore, it would be helpful if you could review the slides as soon as possible and have your report prior to the October 16 meeting.

The National Research Council is the principal operating agency of the National Academy of Sciences and the National Academy of Engineering to serve government and other organizations. The Board on Environmental Studies and Toxicology is responsible to the National Research Council through the Commission on Life Sciences and the Commission on Geosciences, Environment, and Resources.

We highly appreciate your willingness to review the mouse slides for us. With best regards, I am,

Sincerely,

Kulbir S Bakshi

Kulbir S. Bakshi, Ph.D.
Project Director

KSB/cmk

APPENDIX 3

AFIP Response

DEPARTMENT OF DEFENSE
ARMED FORCES INSTITUTE OF PATHOLOGY
WASHINGTON, DC 20306-6000

October 14, 1992

REPLY TO
ATTENTION OF

Kulbir S. Bakshi, Ph.D.
National Research Council
2101 Constitution Ave
Washington, D.C. 20418

Dear Dr. Bakshi:

On 29 September, 1992, in response to your letter dated 24 July, 1992, the Proctor and Gamble mouse fluoride study was reviewed in part at Hazleton Laboratories, Madison, Wisconsin. Present were Drs. Michael Slayter (AFIP), Lent Johnson (AFIP), Steven Weisbrode (The Ohio State University), Byron Boysen (Hazleton Laboratories), and James Maurer (Procter and Gamble). Due to time constraints, our review was limited to a representative sample of bone sections on glass slides from each treatment group. The underlying purpose of this review was to accurately answer the eight specific questions you have posed in the above cited letter. Our response follows:

1. We gather from your letter that the primary lesions of concern are those termed hyperostosis and osteoma. This terminology is correctly used in the study and falls within the limits of time-honored academic definition. As stated in the study, hyperostosis is, 'a term used to describe excessive formation of non-neoplastic bone. The lesion may be focal, multifocal, or diffuse. Morphologically, hyperostoses are characterized by the presence of excessive amounts of woven or lamellar bone or both. Borders between normal bone and areas of hyperostoses cannot usually be distinguished morphologically. In this study, the areas of hyperostoses tended to be bilaterally symmetrical and characterized by irregular deposition of mature lamellar bone primarily in, but not limited to, subperiosteal regions, resulting in excessively thick cortical regions. Although these lesions were also found in other bones, the incidence and severity were much greater for bones of the head.'

Likewise, osteoma is stated as, 'a term used to describe a benign neoplasm arising from osteoblasts. Morphologically, osteomas are usually composed of abundant osteoids/matrix arranged in a spicular pattern and forming spherical masses that have distinct borders that are clearly distinguished from, but attached to, normal bone. The neoplastic bone may be woven or lamellar. These neoplasms are generally distinguished from hyperplastic lesions because osteomas are circumscribed and clinically may continue to grow by expansion after being detected. Osteomas are slow growing expansive lesions and do not metastasize.'

Kulbir S. Bakshi, Ph.D.
Page two

Two additional terms which were used less frequently in the
study, and which may surface in your subsequent discussions are
osteosclerosis and enostosis.   These terms indicated diffuse and
localized ossification of the medullary cavity, respectively.

The definition of other more incidental lesions are also
addressed in the Hazleton report (HLA 81190).

   2.   Human osteomas are often considered neoplasms, but some
authors doubt that they represent true neoplasms.   They are
regarded by some as hamartomas, a general term which can be
applied broadly to a mass of disorganized, mature, specialized
cells or tissue which is indigenous to a particular site, but
present in the wrong proportions.   An accurate definition of
"neoplasm" is surprisingly difficult to establish.   The British
oncologist Sir Rupert Willis provided the best when he wrote, "A
neoplasm is an abnormal mass of tissue, the growth of which
exceeds and is uncoordinated with that of the normal tissues and
persists in the same excessive manner after cessation of the
stimuli which evoked the change."   We agree that the osteomas
reported in this study are virally induced growths but not true
neoplasms; if the evoking virus was removed, the lesion would
persist only as an anomaly in both the controls and the fluoride
treated animals.   Extrapolation to humans is impossible as no
comparable situation is known to occur.

   3.   The osteomas in this study did not appear to result from
the progression of the hyperostoses, nor is the reverse true.

   4.   Inasmuch as no malignant bone tumors were seen among the
many osteomas in the study, we conclude that these osteomas do
not progress to a malignant form.

   5.   True neoplasms do not regress.   Removal of the virus is
a hypothetical question and difficult to address.   Fluoride-
induced changes would eventually regress after removal of the
fluoride; however, it is doubtful that one could appreciate any
substantial regression of the osteoma in the short life span of a
mouse.

   6.   Primary bone neoplasms are rarely multicentric in
animals.   Two notable exceptions are feline osteochondromatosis
(which may not be a true neoplasm) and viral induced tumors of
the mouse.

   7.   Within the experience of the panel, there is no human
counterpart to a fluoride-viral bone perturbation seen in the
mice of this study.

Kulbir S. Bakshi, Ph.D.
Page three

    8. Evidence to support a retrovirus infection consists of
finding numerous C-type retrovirus particles associated with
osteoblasts in all osteomas ultrastructurally examined,
regardless of whether they occurred in control mice or mice
treated with NaF. Retroviruses are known to cause osteomas in
mice. Additionally, the locations, multiplicity and morphologic
features of the osteomas in all groups were consistent with those
associated with virus-induced bone tumors. Attempts to fulfill
Koch's postulate by infecting mice with retrovirus from the study
to demonstrate it would induce osteomas were unsuccessful.
However, the presence of numerous retrovirus particles in all
osteomas examined is highly suggestive of its involvement in the
induction of the osteomas.

Thank you for the opportunity to be of service.

John M. Pletcher, DVM, MPH
Colonel, VC, USA
Chairman, Department of Veterinary Pathology

Michael V. Slayter, DVM, MPVM
Chief, Research Branch
Department of Veterinary Pathology

Lent C. Johnson, M.D.
Orthopedic Research